Finding Fault in California
AN EARTHQUAKE TOURIST'S GUIDE
Susan Elizabeth Hough

2004
Mountain Press Publishing Company
Missoula, Montana

Front cover photograph: The 1992 M7.3 Landers earthquake created this dramatic surface rupture in the Mojave Desert of California.
—MICHAEL RYMER PHOTO, U.S. GEOLOGICAL SURVEY

Library of Congress Cataloging-in-Publication Data
Hough, Susan Elizabeth, 1961-
Finding fault in California : an earthquake tourist's guide /
Susan Elizabeth Hough.
    p. cm.
Includes bibliographical references and index.
ISBN 0-87842-495-4 (pbk. : alk. paper)
  1. Earthquakes—California—Guidebooks. 2. Faults (Geology)—
California—Guidebooks. 3. California—Guidebooks. I. Title.
QE535.2.U6H68 2004
551.8'72'09794—dc22

                                        2004003172

PRINTED IN THE UNITED STATES OF AMERICA

Mountain Press Publishing Company
P.O. Box 2399 • Missoula, Montana 59806
(406) 728-1900

For Sarah, Joshua, and Paul—
three golden natives of a Golden State

Acknowledgments

Before I say anything else, I must start with two confessions. First, to set the record straight, strictly speaking only two of my three children are true natives of the Golden State. My youngest, Paul, is proud to have been born in one of the original thirteen colonies, New Jersey, during the four years of his parents' adult lives during which they lived somewhere other than California. But whereas his siblings have early childhood memories of living in New York, Paul migrated westward in a covered wagon (Subaru) at the tender age of seventeen months, and he remembers no other home than California. According to the spirit if not the letter of the law, he is a native. And although my own childhood roots trace back to a number of points east of the Mississippi River, my roots as a scientist are Californian to the core. I earned my undergraduate degree at the University of California, Berkeley and my Ph.D. at Scripps Institution of Oceanography, a department of the University of California, San Diego. The state has also been my home for all but four of my years as a research scientist.

The second and more relevant confession is that I am not a geologist. The distinction between different fields in the earth sciences may sound like a fine one, but different disciplines can, in fact, be very different. The research that I do is mathematical and computational in nature, typically involving analysis of earthquake waves that seismometers recorded. This is a far cry from the work that geologists do, generally in the field, to investigate faults.

I was able to write this book by listening to, talking to, and reading the papers written by my more geologically inclined colleagues. In this endeavor I have relied on the kindness not of strangers, but of my colleagues and friends: Ramón Arrowsmith, Lisa Grant, Tom Rockwell, Kerry Sieh, Nano Seeber, John Shaw, Aron Meltzner, Clarence Allen, David Hill, David Schwartz, and Michael Rymer. I am especially indebted to four individuals, extraordinary scientists and educators all, who were gracious and patient enough to not only educate me but also to read and give me feedback on chapters of this book. To Sally McGill, Carol Prentice, James Dolan, and Roger Bilham, my most heartfelt gratitude.

A number of my colleagues were also kind enough to provide photographs or figures that appear in these pages, allowing me to present images that were beyond my photographic range in either time or space. My thanks go to Clarence Allen, Rick Sibson, Brian Atwater, John Shaw, Felix Waldhauser, Malcolm Johnson, and Sally McGill. My thanks also go to Bill Murrell, the gracious and intrepid pilot who provided the wings that allowed me to photograph the San Andreas fault from the air.

In sidebars throughout this book, I have highlighted the often ingenious fault-finding methods that my geologically inclined colleagues have developed and applied. These sidebars focus on modern studies, which perhaps leads to an unfortunate neglect of the important fault-finding studies of the past—a deficiency I look forward to remedying in my next book. I am, however, indebted to the individuals whose work is highlighted in this book, especially to the ones (they know who they are) who responded with good humor when I asked if I might put on my reporter's cap to talk to them about their work.

I am also indebted to my editor, Kathleen Ort, for not only finding the faults in my original manuscript but also for offering the perfect suggestions to remedy them. If geologic faults could be so expertly identified and rectified, the world would be a safer place. I also thank Colin Chisholm for smoothing out the remaining kinks in the prose.

Closer to home I have again received a large measure of support from my family, including unwavering encouragement from my father, Jerry Hough, and my husband, Lee Slice, who held the fort while I traipsed hither and yon to find and photograph faults. I wish I could say that my three kids, Sarah, Joshua, and Paul, jumped at the opportunity to join me on these trips and learn about faults, earthquakes, and California geology. Unfortunately, while they do not generally agree on much, they are united in the opinion that faults are duller than, well, dirt. But if they will not be following in their mother's geological footsteps, I am heartened that they have their own passions and are poised to follow their own paths.

As for my own path, I find it interesting to look back and realize that, twenty-odd years ago, earth sciences appealed to me largely for prosaic reasons. Unlike other fields I considered, including mathematics and astronomy, geophysics seemed to offer the possibility of combining mathematical endeavors, meaningful science, and a sane and gainful career with some semblance of balance in my life. The earth sciences might not have been a childhood passion, but they have certainly become an adult one. And although I was not born in the Golden State, California is my home, the land that I love. California is not only one of the best natural laboratories in the world for earthquake science, it is also the most spectacular backyard a person could ask for. I hope I have done it justice in the pages that follow.

1   Introduction:
History Lessons

As every California schoolchild learns in fourth-grade history lessons, if the state's long and fascinating saga has a unifying theme, it can surely be summed up in one word: immigration. From the intrepid wanderers who first arrived via the Bering Strait, to the Spaniards who established the missions along El Camino Real, to the stampede of miners who arrived in the wake of John Marshall's discovery of gold at Sutter's Mill, to the wave of newcomers arriving in recent years from around the Pacific Rim and elsewhere—immigrants have been shaping and reshaping California for thousands of years. This process has created a melting pot arguably unlike any other on earth, an enormously diverse and constantly dynamic culture that is often wonderful, sometimes dreadful, and rarely ever dull.

The rich diversity of California culture seems only fitting when we consider the state from a geologic standpoint. In a geologic sense, the state itself is an amalgamation of immigrants, namely, the detritus of plate tectonics that geologists call accreted terranes. Whereas the central cores of continents have remained intact and stable for hundreds of millions, even billions, of years, continental edges such as California have been not only well shaken but also stirred over time by the ongoing forces of plate tectonics.

The nature of the plate boundary along the western coast of North America has changed over geologic time. Each "wave" of tectonic forces has left its mark on the land as surely as each wave of immigration has left its mark on the culture. The forces of change have left behind a landscape and a culture that are often wonderful, sometimes dreadful, and rarely ever dull.

When fourth-grade social studies classes cover California history, they turn back the clock only so far, at most to the arrival of the first human settlers a few tens of thousands of years ago. Yet to truly understand the state, we must look much farther back in time—about 30 million years farther—to the point that marks the true beginning of modern-day California. This part of the story is not about people but rather about geology. We might suppose that the latter has nothing to do with the former, but we would be wrong.

Long before the first humans arrived in what we now call California, geologic processes gradually crafted the landscape as we know it. Those processes gave birth to the fertile valleys that drew ranchers and farmers, as well as to the idyllic coastal regions that drew millions of late-twentieth-century immigrants hoping to find their piece of the California Dream. In this part of the world, geology has not only shaped history—it *is* history. It is, and forever will remain, a big part of what California is and who Californians are.

To begin, then, at the beginning, we must travel back to a geologic era that postdates the dinosaurs and predates the first humanoids—an era that is, paleontologically speaking, perhaps a little dull. The date was 30 million years before present (BP), give or take a few million years, a point at which a collision occurred. Unlike the meteor impact that scientists now believe wiped out the dinosaurs, this event probably had an inauspicious beginning. It involved the

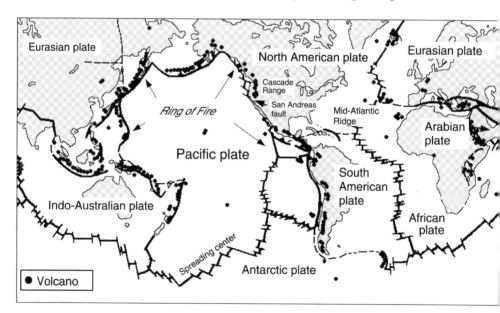

Map of the world with major plate boundaries highlighted. Subduction zones, in which oceanic crust dives beneath continental crust, exist around most of the Pacific Rim, the so-called Ring of Fire, although the San Andreas fault system accommodates transform, or lateral, motion. At spreading centers such as the Mid-Atlantic Ridge, new oceanic crust is created, and the plates move apart. Small circles mark locations of active volcanoes, jagged lines mark spreading centers, and smooth lines mark subduction zones and transform faults.

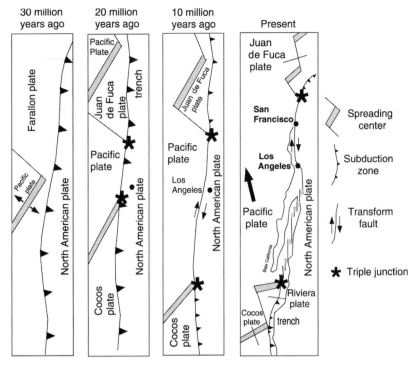

These four panels show the inferred evolution of the boundary system between the Pacific and North American plates, starting with the first encounter between the spreading center and the coast about 30 million years before present and continuing to the present day.

collision of tectonic plates—enormous objects that move more slowly than human hair grows. When plates collide, the consequences are dramatic, but the drama takes millions of years to unfold.

Schoolchildren learn about the theory of plate tectonics at about the same time that they study California history. They learn how the earth's crust is made up of about a dozen major plates that are in continual motion and that most earthquakes occur at the boundaries between those plates. They learn that there are three basic types of plate boundaries: subduction zones, where oceanic crust sinks, or subducts, beneath continental crust; spreading zones, where plates move away from one another and new oceanic crust is created; and transform zones, where plates move past one another laterally.

Basic plate tectonics theory—of the ilk amenable to a fourth-grade curriculum—tends to gloss over some of the more interesting details, including the evolution of plate boundary systems over time. Plate tectonic processes do not evolve in the sense that biological species do, of course, but they do evolve. For example, an ongoing process of subduction might eventually bring one continent careening into another—careening at a speed of 5 centimeters per year, that is—in which case subduction can give way to continental collision.

Prior to 30 million years ago, a spreading center was active in the eastern Pacific Ocean, creating new oceanic crust on both sides of the jagged boundary. Crust created to the east of the spreading center formed what geologists call the Farallon plate. The Farallon plate moved eastward until it encountered and subducted beneath the North American continent. Plate boundaries themselves, though, are typically in motion with respect to each other, and in this case the spreading center was itself migrating eastward. Thirty million years ago, the leading edge of this center collided with the North American landmass. This collision marked the beginning of the end of both the Farallon plate and the process of subduction along North America's western edge. About 25 million years ago (give or take a few million), the Pacific plate thus moved into direct contact with the North American plate, and the complex three-dimensional geometry of the plates gave rise to a lateral relative motion rather than subduction. The San Andreas fault was born.

The transformation of the plate boundary into its modern configuration did not occur overnight. The Farallon plate continued to subduct to the north of where the spreading center first collided with the continent. It took a full 30 million years for the last remnant of subduction to migrate northward to the Oregon border and the San Andreas fault as we know it to define the plate boundary in California. Much of the present-day geography of the state was shaped during that time.

Of course, much of present-day California, including the Sierra Nevada, existed before the San Andreas fault developed. Although the present Sierra Nevada rose and tilted mostly within the past 5 million years, the rocks in that grand range formed 80 million years ago. This book, however, will focus on the more modern tectonic processes that have shaped—and continue to shape—California.

A group of geologists and geophysicists at the University of California at Santa Barbara, led by Tanya Atwater, has developed computer animations to illustrate the evolution of the California landscape from 50 million years ago to the present. Those little movies allow a person to watch a simulation of the state being born. (You can view the movies online at http://www.geol.ucsb.edu/faculty/atwater.)

As many people know, the San Andreas fault is the primary plate boundary between the Pacific and North American plates. It is the boundary along which most of the relative motion has occurred and will continue to occur for the foreseeable geologic future. This impression is consistent with the usual cartoon illustrations of plate tectonics that portray plate boundaries and major faults as one and the same. Reality, however, is more complex. The boundary between the Pacific and North American plates, like all plate boundaries, is a system. While the San Andreas fault is a dominant player in the plate boundary system, it is not the only one. Rather than being a single major fault along which the plates move cleanly past one another, the plate boundary is essentially shearing, or grinding, California into ribbons—and tangled ribbons at that.

To understand the complexity of the plate-boundary system, first consider the geometry of the present-day San Andreas fault. The feature is clearly not linear, but rather bends into a substantial kink as it reaches the Indio–Palm Springs region. Perhaps taking a page from astrophysicists—think Big Bang—geologists know this feature by its highly technical official name, the Big Bend.

The Big Bend exists because the San Andreas fault does not exist in a vacuum. To the east of California, and within eastern California itself, the crust is undergoing a process known as extension, a process by which the crust is slowly stretching and thinning. The origins of this extension are not entirely understood, but most scientists see it as a by-product of the long episode of subduction that defined the plate boundary before the San Andreas fault came into being. According to the theory, that subduction left much of the crust of western North America elevated and the mantle beneath it unusually hot—a combination of circumstances that conspired to produce the current process of extension and the terrain we know as the Basin and Range.

Over the past 20 million years or so, Basin and Range extension has pushed the northern San Andreas fault westward, while the southern segment has experienced no similar shove. This interplay of tectonic processes introduces the kink in the plate-boundary system. Near the Big Bend, the two plates cannot slide past one another smoothly; rather a component of compression, or squeezing, occurs along the bend. This compression affects the southern California landscape in several profound ways, most notably by building mountains.

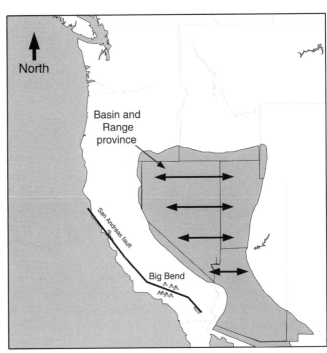

Extension in the Basin and Range province has, according to one theory, created the Big Bend in the San Andreas fault.

Any mountain range on earth is the product of the interplay between competing forces: active tectonic forces that push mountains upward, and more passive erosional forces that wear them down. Both the height and the character of mountain ranges, therefore, reflect their age. The Appalachian Mountains are a good example of an old mountain range, with gently rolling contours and modest heights. But if the Appalachians can be considered geriatric, the mountain ranges of southern California, discussed in detail in chapter 3, must surely be teenagers—active, still growing, and more than a little unruly.

Mountains might represent the most notable manifestation of the plate-boundary complexity, but there are others. Although the present and future evolution of the Pacific–North American plate-boundary system remains the subject of some debate, some earth scientists think that the San Andreas fault will eventually lose its primacy within the system. Over millions—if not tens of millions—of years, the primary plate boundary might well align itself along faults more favorably oriented given the direction the plates are moving, and bypass the pesky Big Bend region altogether. Such faults—faults that, once developed, could align to form a straighter and smoother plate boundary than the present-day San Andreas fault—may exist today.

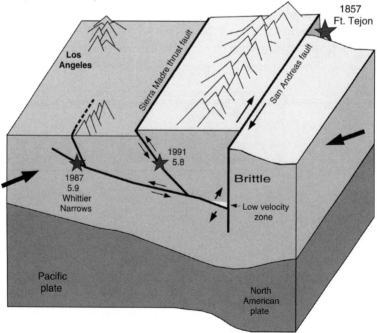

The process by which compression across the San Andreas fault gives rise, so to speak, to mountains. Compression along the Big Bend pushes the Transverse Ranges up along faults such as the Sierra Madre. —AFTER WORK BY GARY FUIS AND OTHERS

According to one theory, some of the most notable recent earthquakes in California reflect a realignment process already underway. Chapter 6 discusses those earthquakes and the ways in which their causative faults have shaped the vast desert regions of southern California.

North of the Big Bend, the plate-boundary system becomes less complex. However, nowhere in the state does the plate boundary collapse to the width of a single narrow fault. The most salient other example of complexity lies, coincidentally, in the state's other major metropolitan region, the San Francisco Bay Area. As chapter 4 discusses, a series of fault splays has shaped this region. The San Andreas itself runs through the San Francisco peninsula, but other important faults branch eastward from the San Andreas. These faults originate south of the bay and run mainly northward through East Bay communities, including Oakland and Berkeley. A veritable spiderweb of faults cuts through the Bay Area, giving rise to complex and distributed seismic hazard.

By the end of chapter 6, this book will have discussed faults, earthquakes, and earthquake hazard in the greater Los Angeles region, the San Francisco Bay Area, central California, and the desert regions of southern California. The chapters include maps and photographs, in most cases with precise GPS (Global Positioning System) coordinates for latitude and longitude, to guide earthquake tourists who are interested in going beyond armchair fault-finding. Color versions of most of the photographs are available over the Web at www.findingfault.com.

These regions, including their offshore environs, combine to form much but not all of the story: the Pacific–North American plate-boundary system encompasses essentially the entire state. This system can be thought of as a complex, dynamic puzzle in which all the pieces not only fit together but also affect one another. The last two chapters of the book, therefore, discuss the remaining puzzle pieces: the eastern Sierran corridor, including the active volcanic system that has threatened Mammoth Lakes; and the nature of the plate boundary outside of the state.

Although not the primary focus of this book, the nature of the plate boundary in both Mexico and the Pacific Northwest is part of the California story. Just as geology provides the framework from which we can understand California's history, the larger plate-tectonic setting provides the context necessary to fully understand California's geology. The astute reader may be wondering, why stop there? Indeed, the earth itself is a puzzle whose pieces are inexorably interrelated. But a book must stop somewhere, and this is not a book about planet Earth. It is about one particular small and wonderful part of the planet, a part that now represents not only a political territory but also a dream—a part whose myriad and spectacular faults easily deserve a book all their own.

2 To Find Them You Have to Know What They Are

Chapter 1 blithely discussed faults with nary a mention of what they are. This leap-before-you-look approach was predicated on the assumption that readers of this book have at least a passing familiarity with the concept of a fault. Most people—particularly most Californians—know that earthquakes occur on structures known as faults. But as is often the case in science, reality belies the seeming simplicity of the concept. Which is to say, it's a fair bet that most readers do not fully understand faults, because even earth scientists still struggle to understand them fully.

Among the questions that remain unresolved about faults are ones as basic as these: How wide are faults? How long/straight are they? Are faults "strong" or "weak"? Are they "wet" or "dry"? To say nothing of the far more complex questions about how faults rupture in earthquakes, which this book will not attempt to tackle in detail.

Active research efforts during the late twentieth and early twenty-first centuries have been shaping a picture of faults themselves. Scientists knew some properties of faults far earlier, of course, such as that they come in three basic types, which correspond, broadly speaking, to the three types of plate boundaries: thrust, normal, and strike-slip. These three kinds of faults accommodate different types of crustal motion, or stress. Squeeze, or compress, a block of crust hard enough and it will eventually break along thrust faults. When thrust faults rupture in earthquakes, the crust becomes thicker, just as a bulldozer creates a higher pile by pushing, or compressing, dirt. Normal faults are the antithesis of thrust faults: they also cut through the crust at an angle, but they accommodate extension, which makes the crust thinner. (Only in bad Hollywood disaster movies do faults open up in great yawning chasms.) Rounding out the trinity are strike-slip faults, which accommodate lateral motion. Nothing moves up or down when a strike-slip fault ruptures. One side of the fault simply moves sideways relative to the other. Scientists say a strike-slip fault is right-lateral if, looking across the fault, the other side moves to the right; if the other side moves to the left, the fault is called left-lateral.

Real-world faults are, not surprisingly, rather more complicated than the simple three-fold taxonomy suggests. Many faults move in not only thrust, normal, or strike-slip motions, but instead incorporate a mixture of either thrust and strike-slip, or normal and strike-slip movements. (Not thrust and normal, of course.) When these so-called oblique-slip faults rupture, they move a certain amount sideways and a certain amount vertically. This represents far more than a taxonomical complication. It can greatly complicate attempts to understand past fault motions based on the features we can observe at the earth's surface.

An additional complication—one that proves critical for an understanding of California's geology—concerns a distinction between different types of thrust faults. Some of them reach the surface and some of them don't. The distinction may appear trivial, but here again there are important implications for understanding the geology and earthquake hazard in California. Thrust faults that don't reach the surface, so-called blind thrusts, will of course disrupt the earth's surface in different ways than thrust faults that do reach the surface. Whereas a regular thrust fault will produce a clean break, or scarp, when it ruptures, a blind thrust fault will warp the overlying crust. A blind thrust fault that terminates relatively deep, say 10 kilometers, will produce a broad, subtle, diffuse zone of warping, whereas a blind fault that ends closer to the surface will produce a more compact zone of deformation. The implications for fault finding become obvious: the

The three main types of faults—strike-slip, thrust, and normal— and a variation of a thrust fault called a blind thrust fault

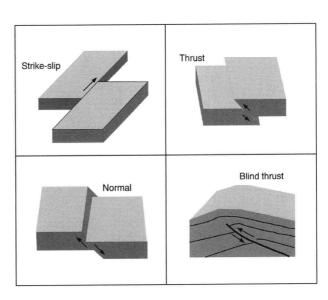

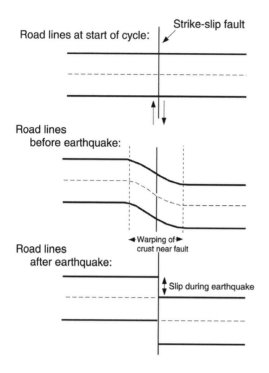

Road lines at start of cycle:

Strike-slip fault

Road lines
before earthquake:

◄ Warping of ►
crust near fault

Road lines
after earthquake:

Slip during earthquake

This cartoon illustrates the tenets of elastic rebound theory. Crust is warped in the vicinity of a locked fault and then moves during an earthquake. The bending of the crust that precedes an earthquake is small, perceptible only by precise geodetic survey methods.

geologist must identify faults based not on ruptures at the surface, but rather on far more subtle features. And not every zone of surface warping has a blind thrust fault beneath it—not by a long shot.

Faults of all types produce earthquakes via the same basic mechanism, known as elastic rebound. As geologist H. F. Reid first proposed the concept shortly after the great 1906 San Francisco earthquake, faults remain locked as forces create pressure, or stress, on and around them. This leads to a buildup of energy, not only on the fault itself but also on both sides of it—to a distance about as large as the fault is deep. When the fault lurches abruptly in an earthquake, that energy is released.

Later in this chapter, and in detail in subsequent chapters, we will explore the ways that faults alter landscapes, using different parts of California as case studies. But let's pause briefly now to address other salient features of faults by returning to the questions posed earlier in this chapter and tackling them one by one.

How wide or thick are faults? The best way to determine the thickness of active faults is to investigate places where current tectonic processes have pushed old faults up to the earth's surface. In such cases, we can examine a fault zone directly. Such lifted faults are not easy to find, but geologists have identified quite a few, and they all reveal the active slip surfaces—the cores, if you will—of faults to be extremely thin, on the order of an inch or less (1 or 2 centimeters). When

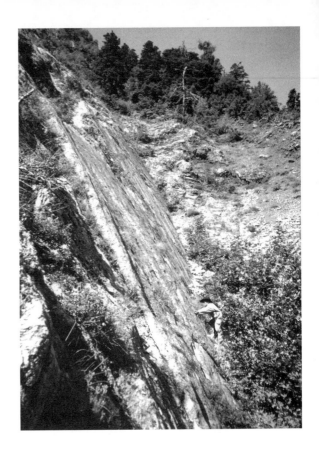

An exposed normal fault near the Aegean Sea on the south shore of the Gulf of Corinth, Greece. The fault zone is several yards wide but in individual earthquakes opposing blocks have slipped past each other on much thinner surfaces, such as the dark band that runs diagonally from the bottom center of the photograph to the top left corner.
—RICK SIBSON PHOTO

gigantic blocks of crust careen past one another in earthquakes, big or small, the so-called slip surfaces that separate them are remarkably narrow.

But this is not the end of the story. Invariably, young fault zones are irregular, made up of many short fault segments generally aligned in the same direction as, but not connected to, one another. A young fault is much like a line of cars imperfectly parked along a curb; an old fault is more like railroad cars linked together into a long and seamless train. Over time, irregular young faults evolve into well-developed old faults as repeated fault movements grind rock near kinks and bends to smithereens. Geologists call this well-pulverized rock gouge. In a mature fault, the gouge zone is typically wider than the narrow slip surface, although it is rarely wider than a few yards.

Panning the camera back farther still, we find that active faults affect the crust to a broader extent than the width of the gouge zone, on the order of 165 to 330 feet (50 to 100 meters)—roughly the length of a football field. Within this fault zone, repeated earthquakes on the fault progressively alter the rock by fracturing and weakening it. Scientists do not entirely understand the process, but the weakening may simply result from powerful, repetitious shaking. In any case, this larger fault zone significantly affects the waves an earthquake

Fault Zones

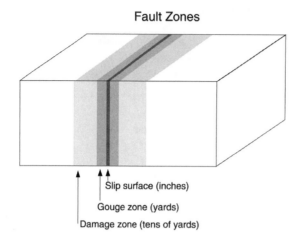

Slip surface (inches)

Gouge zone (yards)

Damage zone (tens of yards)

The multiscale properties of fault zones, including the narrow slip surfaces, wider gouge zone, and even wider zone of damaged rock

generates: energy from a rupture can get trapped within the weaker layer and reverberate, or resonate, producing especially strong shaking. In the late twentieth century, seismologists learned that by observing these waves they could deduce the physical properties of the damage zone, including its width. However, geologic observations strongly suggest that this wide damage zone does not correspond to the actual slip zone.

If we listen to different types of earth scientists discuss fault zones, we might come away thinking about elephants. The proverbial elephant, that is, viewed in entirely different ways by blindfolded individuals who each explore only part of the beast with their hands. Indeed, scientists' views of fault zones have differed sharply over the years depending on the type of data at their disposal. Only in recent years have they begun to appreciate fault zones as complex, multiscale creatures.

Many fault segments collectively form the San Jacinto, Elsinore, and San Andreas faults in southern California.

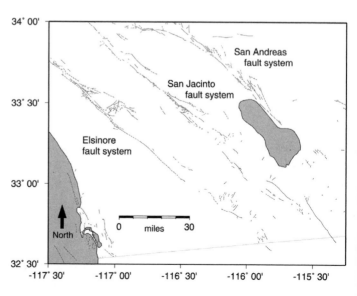

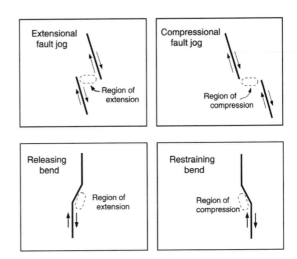

Offsets, or jogs, between successive strike-slip fault segments can give rise to either zones of compression or extension (top). Such zones also exist at bends in faults (bottom).

Indeed, faults are complicated in three dimensions. Moving along the length, or strike, of a fault, we find complexity as well. Continuous, uninterrupted fault strands are far more the exception than the rule when we turn from textbook cartoons to look at the real earth. In the earth, a large fault such as the San Andreas consists of almost innumerable smaller fault pieces or segments. Virtually any fault, big or small, is segmented to some extent.

Fault segments come in various flavors. Commonly, individual segments are each continuous along their trace for only so far, until a small offset separates one segment from the next. The next segment typically begins not directly in front of the last, but slightly to one side of it. This geometry, known as en echelon faulting, leads to interesting consequences when faults rupture. Depending on whether a fault is right- or left-lateral and whether it steps, or jogs, to the right or to the left, fault rupture will create little zones of either compression or extension in the vicinity of the fault jog. Over time, successive ruptures can preserve and build up these features, making them useful for fault finding. Small linear zones of uplift called pressure ridges typically identify compressional fault jogs.

Pressure ridges can also develop along straight fault segments if the fault is not aligned properly to accommodate the geologic forces. For example, the direction of relative plate motion controls forces along the San Andreas fault; the plate motion is uniform but the orientation of the San Andreas fault varies along its length. The Big Bend is essentially a big misalignment, and the San Gabriel Mountains are essentially a big pressure ridge. At many locations elsewhere along the San Andreas, the same theme repeats, but on a much smaller scale. Where faulting produces a vertical step in the landscape—either directly by thrust or normal faulting or as a pressure ridge—geologists call this feature a scarp, which is short for escarpment.

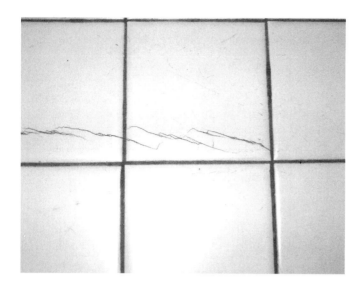

En echelon
fractures in
ceramic tile

Over time, water can collect either behind fault ridges or within the depressions associated with extensional fault bends. The latter are known in the parlance as sag ponds, and they range in size from small ponds to good-sized lakes. In modern times, water management in California has turned some of these natural lakes into reservoirs, typically expanding their size significantly. Because faults are segmented, features such as sag ponds and pressure ridges vary widely in scale, and small-scale features help us investigate the detailed geometry of faults.

The origin of fault segmentation remains an open research issue. In general, scientists think segmentation results from some combination of two factors: 1) complexity in rock type and/or existing topography close to a fault, both of which might make it difficult for ruptures to blast through as straight, unbroken strands; and 2) a more inherent complexity associated with the dynamics of earthquake rupture. The latter idea, while complex in detail, derives a measure of conceptual support from the observation that even simple materials—for instance, ceramic tile on a bathroom floor—tend to fracture in complicated ways.

The segmentation of fault zones raises an interesting question: How badly broken can a fault be and still be considered part of the same fault? The salient issue here is not whether we choose to give disjointed fault segments the same name, but whether they are able to rupture in a single earthquake. This question has critically important implications for modern earthquake hazard assessment, which must relate observed faults in the field with potential future earthquakes. Size matters because the dimensions of the fault rupture control earthquake magnitude. If a fault is only 6 miles (10 kilometers) long, the biggest earthquake that could happen on that fault would be a magnitude 6.0 (give or take); if a fault is 60 miles (100 kilometers) long, an end-to-end rupture would be closer to magnitude

7.5. In both cases, I assume the typical fault depth observed in California, on the order of 9 miles (15 kilometers).

To embark on a brief tangent, throughout this book I use "magnitude" generically and commonly abbreviate it as "M" (M6.5 means magnitude 6.5). The term, however, represents a veritable can of seismological worms (big, fat juicy ones). Original definitions hearken back to the 1930s, to seminal work by Charles Richter and others who developed scales to measure the relative strength of earthquakes. The Richter scale itself is now obsolete; newer scales more faithfully reflect the size of earthquakes, large ones in particular. But all modern magnitude scales are essentially patterned after and designed to overlap with the Richter scale, the mother of all magnitude scales.

Returning to the question at hand, when can segments fairly be considered distinct faults? In the late 1990s, seismologists Ruth Harris and Steven Day developed a sophisticated computer model of fault segments and concluded that earthquakes do not propagate across offsets or fault jogs that are greater than 3 miles (5 kilometers) wide. Subsequent observation of offsets that were and were not ruptured by large earthquakes has generally borne out this result.

But consider the distance for a second: 3 miles. Smaller offsets can and do arrest ruptures, but we cannot count on an earthquake to stop at an offset unless it is a full 3 miles wide. That's pretty remarkable considering that a law-abiding driver on the freeway would need a full three minutes to traverse the same distance.

Thus we arrive at a picture of faults that is very far removed from the cartoon lines of the figure on page 9. Faults are, quite literally, complicated in every direction.

Moving along to the next seemingly simple question, are faults strong or weak? The question might appear simple to the point of triviality, for one of the very first things beginning geology students learn about faults is that they are preexisting zones of weakness in the crust. A zone of weakness—a fracture, a fault—is surely weak.

If faults are weak, though, why do they stay locked until they rupture in earthquakes? Imagine slicing a block of wood in two and applying sideways pressure on both sides of the block. The two halves would slide steadily against each other. But except for a small handful of cases, faults do not exhibit the steady, ongoing motion that geologists term creep. Instead, the two sides of a fault remain motionless, or locked, by virtue of the friction between them. Geologists define a coefficient of friction to describe the overall strength of faults, with a minimum value of zero (no friction) and a maximum value of one. A coefficient of friction in the neighborhood of 0.3 indicates a weak fault; a value up around 0.8, a strong one. And different studies have inferred values that span this range.

It is very difficult to measure the strength of faults directly. Instead seismologists draw inferences based on indirect observations such as the orientation of earthquake ruptures along minor faults in the neighborhood of a major fault. Such calculations involve not only fairly subtle theoretical considerations but also extremely difficult numerical calculations. Toward the end of the 1990s, different scientists (well-respected, all) interpreted a single set of observational results to yield diametrically opposite conclusions about fault strength.

In recent years, some scientists have argued that the answer to this conundrum can be found by considering fault geology and earthquake physics together. Their reasoning involves considering the energy associated with earthquake ruptures. When a fault moves, stored energy is released—just as the snap of our fingers releases the energy stored by pushing them together before they snap. And not unlike the case of snapping fingers, earthquakes release energy in different forms. In both cases, a small percentage of the energy radiates as waves (sound waves and/or shear waves) while most of the stored energy drives the actual motion of the objects in motion (fingers on the one hand, so to speak; blocks of rock on the other). However, in both cases a certain amount of energy is associated with more subtle processes. Forcing our fingers past each other under pressure generates an imperceptible but finite amount of heat; a certain amount of energy also disrupts the very outermost layer of cells (or at least the dirt) on our skin. So, too, are heat and damage associated with fault ruptures.

In fact, some scientists argue heat is the key to understanding faults. Theoretical calculations show that the amount of heat associated with earthquake ruptures depends on the thickness of the rupture zone. The thinner the fault, the greater the heat produced locally in the earthquake. With faults as thin as some of those observed in the field, calculations predict that if faults were not weak, earthquake ruptures would generate enough heat to melt rock. The idea of melting rock is not totally outlandish. Scientists have observed evidence—geologic detritus—of melting in the form of pseudotachylites, small bits of rock that show signs of having melted and then recooled. The primary source of pseudotachylites is the impact craters from large meteors, such as the one that caused the extinction of the dinosaurs 65 million years ago. Pseudotachylites are found only rarely in fault zones, suggesting that rock melting does not occur commonly during earthquakes. Therefore, if faults are thin and earthquakes do not melt rock when they rupture, then they must be weak. Or so the argument goes.

If this reasoning is correct, the next question is, how do faults stay weak? It is one thing for a fault to be weak near the earth's surface, but quite another a few miles deep, where everything exists in dense-pack conditions. The extreme pressure of the overlying rock essentially translates into lateral pressure as well. One possible answer relates to the final question posed at the beginning of this chapter: Are faults wet or dry? If fault zones somehow trap or hold water, then the fluid may serve as a lubricant that maintains a low coefficient of friction (that is, a weak fault). Indeed, geologic evidence shows a pervasive presence of water in fault zones, both deep in the crust and near the earth's surface.

The obvious question then is, why do faults stay locked if they are lubricated and therefore weak? Earth science does not yet have a complete answer to this question, or to other related questions discussed here. One possibility, however, is that fluids exist only in isolated pockets along fault zones, and it is within these pockets that earthquake ruptures nucleate and gain enough steam to produce large earthquakes.

But let me now pose a different sort of question: Who cares if faults are thick or thin, strong or weak, wet or dry? Why bother discussing them at such length here? The answer to this question is as multilayered as fault zones themselves. First, any self-respecting book about faults in California needs to pause to first consider the question, what is a fault, anyway? Faults are indeed interesting creatures, complex beyond what a beginning earth-science student can possibly imagine. Even at the dawn of the twenty-first century, some of the hottest (so to speak) unresolved questions in the earth sciences concern the detailed physical and mechanical properties of faults. Finally, as the title of this chapter implies, it is difficult to find faults if we don't have a clear sense of what we are looking for. Furthermore, finding faults is far more than an interesting exercise for either the scientist or the itinerant earthquake tourist. The fruits of geologists' fault-finding efforts provide essential input for assessing modern earthquake hazard.

Finding faults in California is a legal as well as a scientific matter. The Alquist-Priolo Act, passed in 1972 following the Sylmar earthquake of 1971, was designed to make sure that dwellings not be built on the traces of active faults. This then begs the question: Exactly what is an "active" fault? The Act defined an active fault as one that had ruptured in the last 11,000 years—a time geologists call the Holocene epoch. The California Geological Survey (formerly the California Division of Mines and Geology) assembles and maintains the maps of the state's active fault zones, now available in both print and CD format. This database is, however, very much a work in progress, and information about faults—and the most recent earthquakes on them—continues to be assembled.

However, once we understand what we are looking for, we quickly understand why finding faults—especially secondary faults whose features are less than spectacular—can be such a difficult game. The odds of making detailed surface observations of faults barely an inch (1 to 2 centimeters) thick are slim to none. However, we can observe narrow slip zones at the surface if an earthquake rupture is fresh. Additionally, in a small percentage of cases, especially where a fault cuts very solid rock, a narrow slip zone will remain distinct for many years—hundreds of thousands of years in some cases. But for the most part, erosional processes at the earth's surface are not kind to features this small. Within the

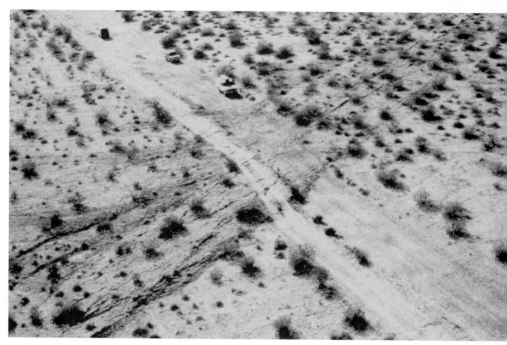

Zone of distributed fault rupture associated with the 1992 Landers, California, earthquake. At the surface, the rupture zone encompassed a zone some 46 feet (15 meters) across. —S. BRYANT PHOTO, CALIFORNIA DEPARTMENT OF MINES AND GEOLOGY

span of a decade—barely the blink of an eye in geologic time—much of the evidence of a fault rupture can be dramatically obscured.

It doesn't help matters that rocks close to the surface are not usually very solid to begin with. The ground might look solid—and it certainly feels solid enough if we land on it the wrong way—but to an earth scientist it is typically quite soft. To a seismologist, El Capitan in Yosemite National Park is hard rock, the foothills in the Los Angeles area are soft rock, and sedimentary deposits within the Los Angeles basin are barely rock at all. If we measure the speed of earthquake waves through the different types of rock, we find dramatic differences: waves travel far faster in hard rock than in soft rock, and faster in soft rock than in sediment.

The kind of rock at the earth's surface also makes a difference in the nature of earthquake ruptures. Earthquakes invariably initiate deep in the crust, usually at least 3 miles (5 kilometers) down. At such depths, the enormous pressure of the overlying material will compact any sort of rock and render it both hard and strong. A large earthquake rupture will propagate outward from its point of origin, its hypocenter, sideward and usually upward along the fault plane. In the sideward direction, the rupture encounters consistently hard rock, but as it moves upward it runs into progressively softer material. At a certain point even the most energetic rupture cannot cut cleanly through soft rock, similar to the way a crisp tear in a piece of paper won't stay crisp when it encounters a soggy patch.

When a rupture encounters soft rock or sediment, one of two things generally happens. In some cases the upward progression of the rupture may cease altogether. This sort of damping may be one of the reasons some thrust faults never reach the surface. In other cases the rupture might reach the surface as a complex, distributed zone of fractures rather than a thin, clean break. In either case the surface manifestation of even a large earthquake rupture can be greatly obscured (but still recognizable) even before any weathering processes begin.

The business of finding a fault, in the sense of identifying the narrow active slip zone itself, might seem a little like looking for the proverbial needle in a haystack—except that in this case the needle degrades quickly, becoming more haylike with each passing rainstorm. Many faults do, however, disrupt the landscapes in significant ways. Viewed through the keen eye of the trained geologist, many of the needles look more like pitchforks.

Still, one reason it took scientists so long to fully quantify the width of faults is that the actual slip surfaces, or planes, are not always easy to find. If we seek to understand the nature of earthquake rupture at depth, we need to examine slip surfaces that have been exhumed from deep within the crust—but without significant alteration. The field geologists who have documented the narrowness of slip zones have traveled to the far ends of the earth to find enough examples from which to draw conclusions, and they reached these conclusions only in the waning years of the twentieth century.

Fortunately for those interested in both geology and seismic hazard, macroscopic properties of fault zones can provide a great deal of important information. By macroscopic properties, I mean the large-scale effect that active faults have on the earth's landforms. We can observe these properties relatively easily for many different types of faults, and in many different types of rock. And it is possible to make at least qualitative inferences from our observations without any sort of specialized tools or analytic methods. Even though the basic theory describing the buildup and release of stress on faults was not established until the 1906 San Francisco earthquake, scientists recorded observations of large-scale fault features well before this time. For instance, the great 1857 Fort Tejon earthquake produced a lateral tear in the earth hundreds of miles long. The individuals who observed it did not know about the San Andreas fault—it hadn't even been named yet—much less understand the relationship between the fault and the plate boundary. But, as we'll discuss in chapter 3, they could, and did, describe its effects. Similarly, observers documented a large earthquake that tore through the Owens Valley in eastern California in 1872, as well as the great 1891 Mino-Owari earthquake in Japan.

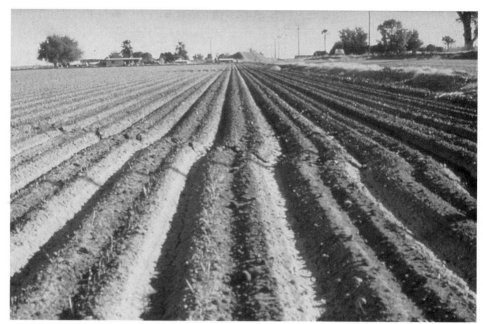

Offset of cultivated fields near El Centro, California, following the M7.1 Imperial Valley earthquake of October 15, 1979. Scientists can infer the amount of offset, or slip, directly from the offset of the rows, although they must take the precise fault orientation into account. —G. REAGOR PHOTO, U.S. GEOLOGICAL SURVEY, DISTRIBUTED BY NOAA/NGDC

So what do faults do? A single earthquake rupture will translate blocks of crust relative to each other according to the style of the fault—a straightforward enough idea. But the evidence that an earthquake leaves behind depends critically on the local setting. If a strike-slip rupture tears through a flat desert, as they have been wont to do in recent years in California, even in the immediate aftermath of the earthquake we can observe only, at best, cracks in the ground. Looking at cracks in a sea of tumbleweeds, it is tough or even impossible to determine how far the sides of the fault moved relative to each other. When such earthquakes happen, geologists try to find reference features that cut across the fault linearly before the earthquake struck.

When movement along a fault breaks such a linear feature, it creates a pair of reference features, so-called piercing points, that reflect the motion of the fault. Natural features—most commonly stream channels—can create piercing points. Once a fault ruptures across a stream, the pair of (offset) points where the stream intersects the fault are the piercing points. Nowadays, however, human-made features and structures commonly provide the best source of data. Roads, fences, sidewalks—any linear feature—is a potential pair of piercing points. Even in the

Even in the sparsely populated deserts of southern California, such linear features are generally rife—or if not rife, at least present to some extent.

Earth scientists use offsets in human-made structures to infer the amount of movement, or slip, in an earthquake. If more than one earthquake bisected a feature, its offset would reflect the cumulative effect of all of the ruptures. However, few if any human-made structures are old enough to have been disrupted by more than one earthquake. People also tend to fix things, such as fences and roads, when something like an earthquake rips them out of kilter. Human-made features, therefore, provide information almost exclusively about individual earthquake ruptures.

To study a longer record of earthquake ruptures, geologists must rely on natural features that earthquakes have progressively altered. Again, the feature that scientists most commonly use in this type of study is the stream channel. The inherent properties of stream channels make them handy tools for geologists. They exist where there is sufficient topography (in mountains or hills) and by definition they run downhill. Channels usually meander, particularly on gently sloping surfaces, but channels on steeper slopes cut a more linear downslope path. A hillside, then, is typically cut intermittently along its face by mostly straight lines running downhill.

Strike-slip faults, meanwhile, commonly run along the bases of mountains or hills perpendicular to the channels. Therefore, when they rupture they cut through the stream channels. Later chapters discuss the detailed manifestation of the San Andreas fault in different parts of California—how it has successively ruptured stream channels, how it has shaped the landscape, and what we can learn from geologic field observations. In particular, by excavating and carefully investigating sediments in some stream channels, geologists can now develop chronologies of prehistoric earthquakes on faults, a subfield of earth science called paleo-seismology. Geologists Malcolm Clark, Lloyd Cluff, Jim McCalpin, and others conducted pioneering work in paleoseismology in the late 1960s and early 1970s. The field burgeoned in the mid- to late 1970s with extensive investigations of the San Andreas fault and Wasatch Front (Utah) faults by geologists Kerry Sieh, David Schwartz, Kevin Coppersmith, and others.

Thrust faults and normal faults, on the other hand, affect the landscape in less subtle ways by creating vertical offsets, or scarps. We might imagine that such offsets are easier to study than are lateral motions because they form obvious stair steps. Such steps do exist throughout California; the chapters that follow will include many photographs of conspicuous scarps that delineate the paths of thrust faults across the landscape.

Unfortunately, two factors greatly complicate the life of the geologist who wants to study thrust faults. The first, introduced earlier in this chapter, is that some thrust faults do not reach the surface at all. The second complicating factor is that the process of erosion can quickly batter even substantial fault scarps.

By virtue of their inherent geometry, fault scarps are destined to lose their sharp edges. When a thrust fault ruptures, the so-called hanging block moves upward, forming an overhanging cliff that is not very stable. Gravity and erosion conspire to modify this unnatural geometry, sometimes with amazing speed. The sharp edge of the hanging block is inevitably the first casualty, slumping to form a feature called a colluvial wedge. Over time, the feature will become smoother still. In the 1980s, seismologist (not actor) Tom Hanks showed that the evolution of fault scarps could be described mathematically, with the offset becoming progressively smoother in time. By measuring the smoothness of an offset, scientists can estimate, at least roughly, the age of a fault scarp. An abrupt stair step must be relatively young; a smoother offset, relatively old.

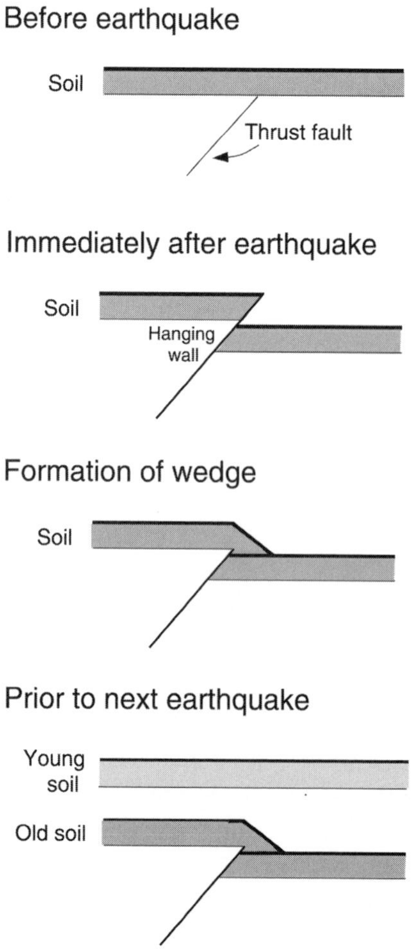

Before earthquake

Soil

Thrust fault

A fresh thrust-fault scarp (second from top) can collapse to form a so-called colluvial wedge (third from top). Over time, younger soils can bury such a fault feature (bottom).

Immediately after earthquake

Soil

Hanging wall

Formation of wedge

Soil

Prior to next earthquake

Young soil

Old soil

We can identify thrust faults—those that are not blind—as smoothed stair steps that cut more or less linearly across the landscape. Unfortunately, from the point of view of fault finding, not every geologic stair step is a thrust fault. In particular, stream channels also cut linear incisions through the crust that can be like stair steps. We can easily distinguish a modern stream channel from a fault scarp, but an ancient stream channel—particularly one that has been differentially eroded—can look a lot like a fault. However, stream channels flow downhill, so a stair step that trends across a hillside rather than down a hill cannot be the wall of a stream channel and is a likely candidate for a fault scarp.

Fortunately, another feature besides sharp geometric angles distinguishes many thrust faults: over time, earthquakes on thrust faults bring different types of rock into contact with one another. If we observe one type of rock pushed up over another type of rock, it's a fair bet that a fault lies between the two (although more typically thrust faults push older rocks over younger ones).

Geologists have developed other ingenious methods to investigate blind and non-blind thrust faults. If a thrust fault ruptures near a coastline, the land can rise abruptly, sometimes defining so-called marine terraces marked by stair-step offsets. In these situations, the former shoreline is suddenly elevated above its former position. Scientists can identify marine terraces by their characteristic geometry as well as by the presence of seashells and corals. A primary challenge of interpreting such terraces can be the timing of, rather than the identification of, uplifts. In some cases, scientists can use detailed analysis of marsh pollens to unravel the history of a coastal region; in other cases, they can use archeological artifacts. By identifying fault-related marine terraces and dating their uplift, scientists have been able to infer the timing of earthquakes and even the existence of previously unknown faults.

Normal faults are like thrust faults in reverse. By virtue of a normal fault's geometry, though, its initial slope is steep but not vertical or overhanging. However, normal faults exist where extensional forces are pulling the crust apart. The active tectonic processes in California are primarily compressional and lateral. Normal faults are therefore relatively rare beasts in California. They exist in abundance, however, in the Basin and Range province east of the state as well as in the eastern part of California.

Entire books can be, and have been, written on the subject of geomorphology, the study of the characteristics and development of landforms. Entire books can be, and have been, written on the geology and mechanics of faults. This chapter has provided but a brief introduction to both subjects. I hope it will provide sufficient background to allow us to continue in our quest—to find fault in California.

3 Finding Fault in Los Angeles

There is an old joke that perhaps sums up the difference between the prevailing culture and self-image of the San Francisco Bay Area and that of Los Angeles. If you want to start a conversation in San Francisco, the joke begins, you say something bad about Los Angeles; if you want to start a conversation in Los Angeles, you say something bad about Los Angeles. Even confirmed Angelenos are typically happy to admit that their hometown is something of a mess—a diverse, sprawling, unruly mess. The problem is not that there is no "there" there. The problem is that there is "there" everywhere: the laid-back, quintessentially Californian beach communities; the richly multicultural valleys; the fabled history of Hollywood; the mountains so close and untamed that black bears and mountain lions wander down to nosh on fallen backyard avocados and small family pets.

Southern California's geologic and geographic diversity is scarcely incidental to its richly diverse culture. Rather, the two are inexorably intertwined. Why is the greater Los Angeles metropolitan region the mess—or maybe we can call it the marvelous patchwork quilt—that it is? The answer is clear to commuters and earth scientists alike: because several prominent mountains cut across the region and divide it into valleys and basins. Just as the separate islands of the Galapagos allowed species to evolve independently, a measure of geographical isolation significantly bolsters the odds of developing a unique regional culture. It is not only a matter of physical isolation, either. The mountain ranges of southern California define markedly different climate zones as well. In a very real sense, the temperament of each region within greater Los Angeles is fundamentally shaped by its geology.

In chapter 1 we explored the origins of the forces now acting on the mountain ranges in the greater Los Angeles area—namely, the broad zone of compression

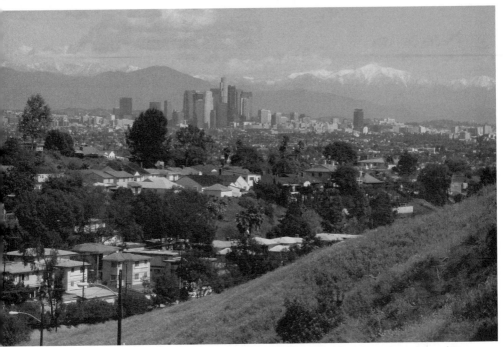

The San Gabriel Mountains, part of the Transverse Ranges, rise over downtown Los Angeles. In the distance, snow-capped Mount Baldy reaches a height of 8,600 feet (2,620 meters). The Sierra Madre fault cuts through the northern San Gabriel Valley and runs along the base of the mountains. (34 00.16N 118 20.94W)

associated with the Big Bend in the San Andreas fault. This zone stretches from well east of San Bernardino all the way to the coast near Santa Barbara and consists of a swath of mountains known collectively as the Transverse Ranges.

The Transverse Ranges earned their name by being, well, transverse in orientation. Most of California's mountains, most notably the vast Sierra Nevada, run roughly north-south. On a topographic map of the state, the Transverse Ranges stand out like a sideways thumb, but we can understand their origins and their orientation in the context of the plate-boundary evolution discussed in chapter 1. As the San Andreas fault established itself, in some cases fragments of the North American plate broke off and became part of the Pacific plate. Other fragments of crust were buffeted in the melee, including several slivers in southern California that the fault caught and rotated clockwise into their present sideways orientation. These slivers became mountain ranges that rose progressively by subsequent (and ongoing) forces of plate tectonics.

A series of seismological investigations in the 1980s and 1990s has revealed that the Transverse Ranges extend down as well as up. That is, the mountains have a unique underpinning—also eloquently known in geologic circles as a drip—of dense rock that has started to sink as a result of ongoing compression. Most mountain ranges have roots—thickened continental crust at depth that, by virtue of being less dense than mantle rocks, buoys the elevation against gravity. The drip beneath the Transverse Ranges is different; it is more dense than surrounding rock. This drip can only be imaged using sophisticated seismological investigations that employ earthquake waves to create the geologic equivalent of a CAT scan. The upward manifestation of the mountains, meanwhile, is anything but subtle.

For many residents of southern California, the Transverse Ranges are a pretty backdrop—at times even snowcapped—and a convenient outdoor playground replete with hiking trails, campsites, ski hills, and wildlife. But the influence of these mountains is far more profound than we might imagine. Large mountain ranges force incoming air upward, where it thins and cools by about 3.5 degrees Fahrenheit per 1,000 feet of elevation. Colder air is, in turn, less able to hold water. In southern California, prevailing winds blow in from the ocean and push eastward, so the wetter, windward side of the Transverse Ranges lies south and west of the mountains. The drier leeward side, meanwhile, lies to the north and east. Thus do the Transverse Ranges separate vast desert regions of southern California from the greater Los Angeles metropolitan area.

Anyone who has spent time in the Los Angeles area knows that, extraordinarily diverse climates exist here in proximity to one another. The weather varies dramatically as we move inland from the coast, and to some extent as we move up and down the coast as well. To understand how the climate changes away from the coast, we must first understand the coastal climate itself. Along any coast, the ocean acts as an effective insulator. Because water heats and cools more slowly than land or air, an ocean will buffer the climate of immediately adjacent coastal regions. Off the coast of southern California, the ocean temperatures are especially cool (for their latitude) because of the overall circulation patterns in the eastern Pacific Ocean (a happenstance that, incidentally, spares Californians from adding hurricanes to their list of potential natural disasters—the waters offshore of the state being too cold to sustain these killer storms).

The presence of the ocean buffers the coastal climate in several ways, including through the creation of fog. Cold ocean water helps chill the air, and when the air above the ocean drops to a certain temperature, water condenses in the air to form ground-hugging clouds, or fog. Offshore of southern California, the ocean water and, therefore, the ocean air are typically cool, which leads to the formation of a thick fog bank known as a marine layer. When the onshore air temperature cools at night, fog can form and push in from the ocean. The extent of this push depends in large part on the barometric pressure over the western United States. Large lobes of high pressure keep the fog at bay, while low pressure systems allow it to make greater inroads.

In the morning, the sun warms the onshore air, eventually causing the fog in the inland marine area to burn off. The closer to the ocean, the greater is the buffering effect of the water itself and the slower the daytime warming. Farther inland, the marine layer typically burns off early in the day. Without the clouds to shield the rays of the sun, the inland temperature rises quickly. As southern California beachgoers know only too well, hot inland temperatures are no guarantee of warm and sunny conditions at the beach.

Proximity to the ocean accounts for much of the small-scale variation in climate across the Los Angeles area, but some of the variation is also associated with mountains—mountains that are smaller than the Transverse Ranges but still large enough to affect weather. We'll investigate some of these mountains and their effects later in this chapter. In general, as we move eastward from the coast to the foot of the mountains in southern California, we find a transition from a temperate coastal climate to a more arid one. The Transverse Ranges, meanwhile, represent the demarcation line that separates the entire greater Los Angeles region from the true desert that lies on the leeward side of the mountains.

Within the Los Angeles area, the climatic complexity reflects an interplay between land and sea—between the ocean and an expanse of continental crust that dramatic plate-tectonic forces continue to shape and reshape. And climate variability is part of what makes the different parts of the greater Los Angeles region as wonderfully distinct as they are—this in addition to the fundamental geographic boundaries that the region's myriad mountains and hills form. Let's now discuss specific regions within this grand geologic melange, embarking on a fault tour beginning with the eastern edge of the greater Los Angeles metropolitan area and moving progressively westward toward the coast.

The Inland Empire

San Bernardino and its environs are the easternmost cities that the Big Bend in the San Andreas fault influences. The so-called Inland Empire, however, enjoys (well, not really) the unique distinction of also being at a geologic crossroads. The San Andreas fault defines the northern edge of the San Bernardino Basin, and the San Jacinto fault—one of the largest and most active secondary faults in the state—defines the western edge of this basin. By virtue of its proximity to both faults (as well as to the Cucamonga fault, which forms the eastward end of the Sierra Madre fault system), San Bernardino faces a level of earthquake hazard that is high even by California standards.

Although the confluence of major faults positions the Inland Empire for something of a double whammy, the region's big problem is the future proverbial Big One on the San Andreas. Over the last few million years, continued right-lateral motion on the San Andreas fault effectively created two mountain ranges out of one. Through the Big Bend region, the Transverse Ranges to the north

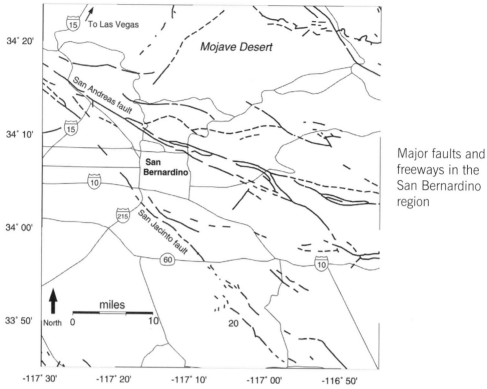

Major faults and freeways in the San Bernardino region

of the fault have moved progressively eastward relative to those parts of the ranges to the south of the fault. To the east of the junction between the San Andreas and San Jacinto faults, we now find the San Bernardino Mountains, home to the popular resort communities of Lake Arrowhead and Big Bear. To the west of the fault juncture, west of San Bernardino, we find the San Gabriel Mountains, which we'll look at later in this chapter. Both the San Gabriel and the San Bernardino Mountains mark an important geographical boundary in the greater Los Angeles region. For the most part, the densely populated urban sprawl of southern California ends where the mountains begin. Throughout most of this area, we enter National Forest land almost as soon as we enter the mountains; in some parts, we encounter terrain that is inhospitable by virtue of its rugged topography and ever-present fire danger.

Although desert communities north of the Transverse Ranges (see chapter 6) are growing, their populations still pale in comparison to the urban regions south of the mountains. And in bisecting and dividing the Transverse Ranges, the San Andreas fault has not been evenhanded in meting out hazard for the densely populated urban areas along the southern mountain front. East of San Bernardino, the San Andreas fault skirts the south side of the mountains, whereas to the west it runs along their northern edge.

To understand why this happenstance poses a particularly acute problem for San Bernardino, we must understand the three primary factors that determine how much the ground will shake at any one location during an earthquake. First, and most obviously, ground shaking will depend on the magnitude of the earthquake. Second, and perhaps equally obvious, shaking will depend on the distance to the rupturing fault. Just as ripples in a pond diminish in amplitude as they spread into ever-greater circles, so too do earthquake waves diminish in the earth's crust as they move away from the source. The third factor that influences the severity of shaking is the type of rock in the shallow crust beneath each location. Where the rock is soft, such as young and therefore poorly consolidated sedimentary rock or loose sediment, shaking is generally amplified compared to that experienced on harder rock such as granite.

In terms of ground shaking, San Bernardino faces a triple whammy. The fault that defines its northern boundary ruptures in extremely large earthquakes—up to and including the M8.0 earthquakes commonly assumed to represent the Big One in California. Moreover, these earthquakes will rupture extremely close to the population centers, and they will occur quite frequently—perhaps every one hundred to three hundred years on average. If this weren't bad enough, most of the population of the greater San Bernardino region is concentrated in the San Bernardino Basin, which is filled with—you guessed it—soft sediment. Frequent

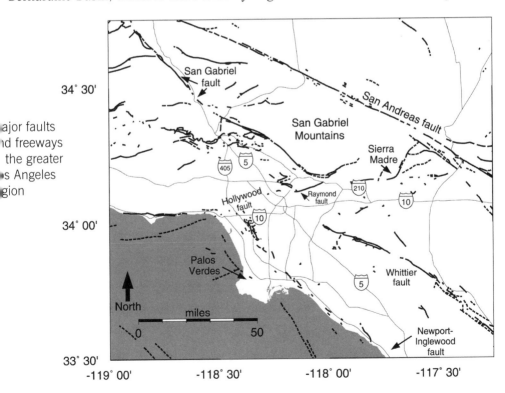

ajor faults
d freeways
the greater
s Angeles
gion

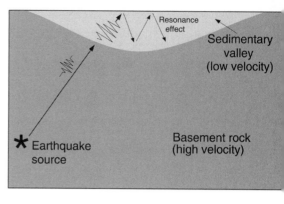

The amplification of seismic waves in sedimentary layers, such as those that we find in valleys of southern California. Waves encounter sedimentary layers, which have lower seismic velocities than hard rock such as granite, and their amplitudes increase—just as a pan of Jell-O wiggles more than a pan of brownies in response to the same disturbance. Waves can also become trapped within sedimentary layers, leading to a pronounced resonance effect that amplifies waves at certain frequencies.

large earthquakes, close faults, soft soils—in terms of earthquake hazard, it doesn't get much worse.

Yet awareness and investigation of earthquake hazard in the Inland Empire has lagged behind that of the Los Angeles area. For example, whereas by the end of the twentieth century, seismologists had developed detailed models of the subsurface structure of the Los Angeles Basin and used those models to predict shaking from future large earthquakes, similar investigations had only just begun for the San Bernardino at that time. Two main reasons may account for the relative inattention given to the Inland Empire: its smaller population, and the absence of large earthquakes in the region in recent times. The last big earthquake to rupture the San Andreas fault near San Bernardino was the great 1857 Fort Tejon earthquake.

The Fort Tejon rupture extended from Parkfield to Wrightwood, near Cajon Pass. We'll examine the Fort Tejon earthquake in chapter 5, but Cajon Pass itself merits a bit of discussion here. For many southern Californians, Cajon Pass is the gateway to one of the southland's favorite getaways: Las Vegas, Nevada. On a given weekend, tens of thousands of Angelenos make the four-hour drive up I-15 from San Bernardino to Las Vegas (and on Sunday nights, the eight-hour drive home). So large is the weekend exodus (and subsequent return) that traffic jams are a familiar sight on the stretch of I-15 between San Bernardino and Barstow—a segment that passes through an expanse of desert where one would expect to find jackrabbits rather than bumper-to-bumper traffic. Yet, onerous as the drive may be, it could easily be worse. Had the San Andreas fault not separated the San Bernardino and San Gabriel Mountains, there would be no Cajon Pass. The drive from Los Angeles to Las Vegas would either be much longer or far more circuitous.

Of course, without the San Andreas fault there would be no mountains in the first place, which should lessen the debt of gratitude southland drivers owe the fault. The mountains also corral the smog, limiting the extent to which the region shares its bumper crop of air pollution with the rest of the planet. Furthermore, without the mountains, there would be no windward side of the mountains— no buffering effect on the climate and no increase in precipitation to help quench the enormous water needs of southern California. Without the mountains the greater Los Angeles area would be not only flatter, but also hotter and more arid. If suddenly granted a proverbial three wishes, Angelenos would, therefore, be ill-advised to wish away the San Andreas fault and the Transverse Ranges.

Returning to I-15 and Cajon Pass, then, heading northward away from San Bernardino, the interstate makes a pronounced westward bend along Cajon Creek just where I-15 merges with I-215. From there, I-15 parallels the fault, which runs just east of the interstate. The freeway crosses the fault several miles farther ahead, between the Kenwood and Cleghorn exits. A seemingly innocuous canyon, Lone Pine Canyon, veers away to the left (northwest) from I-15 about 4 miles north of the I-15/I-215 merge. The slow but inexorable motion of the San Andreas fault carved the passageway of Lone Pine Canyon.

Geologically speaking, the region around Cajon Pass is fairly complicated, not only because of the mountains but also because of the juncture between the San Andreas and San Jacinto faults. And, returning (finally) to the year 1857, this complexity very likely controlled the termination of the great Fort Tejon earthquake. Having probably begun in central California near Parkfield, the 1857 temblor ruptured approximately 240 miles (400 kilometers) of the San Andreas fault before coming to a stop at Cajon Pass. The earthquake predated Reid's elastic rebound theory by fully fifty years, but the effects of this great earthquake were apparent even to the untrained eye of *Visalia Iron Age* editor Stephen Barton. Shortly after the 1857 temblor, Barton wrote, "The line of disturbing force followed the Coast Range some seventy miles west of Visalia and thence out on the Colorado Desert. This line was marked by a fracture of the earth's surface, continuing in one uniform direction for a distance of two hundred miles. The fracture presented an appearance as if the earth had been bisected and the parts had slipped upon each other." Not a bad description from a writer born a century before the development of plate-tectonics theory. Based largely on the inferred length and slip of the fault, seismologists estimate the magnitude of the quake at 7.8 to 7.9.

The year 1857 predates more than modern seismology. It also very nearly predates the existence of southern California as a region populated by humans of European descent. There were people in the region at the time, but only a bare handful compared to the tens of millions who reside there now. Los Angeles was home to approximately 4,000 residents at the time; Fort Tejon itself was far smaller still. The 1857 earthquake cracked houses in Los Angeles and caused more sub-stantial damage to buildings at Fort Tejon, but, by virtue of the sparse population, the earthquake claimed only two lives.

As awful as great earthquakes are, there is something to be said for having a major disaster in an area's not-too-distant past, because where earthquakes are concerned, familiarity begets awareness. For example, in San Bernardino, which lies at arguably the single most dangerous fault nexus in California, scientific investigations have unfortunately lagged behind those of areas hit more recently by large earthquakes.

Because of the paucity of recent earthquakes, dramatic and clear evidence of faulting is hard to come by in the Inland Empire. Fault features tend to be large-scale and, therefore subtle when viewed from ground level. We can, however, find dramatic fault features. In the city of Highland, just east of San Bernardino, the San Andreas fault creates a clear ridge that crosses Church Street, just north of Highland Avenue. To the west of Church Street the fault zone is identifiable by the standard 50-foot-wide no-build zone. Luxury homes have sprung up in recent years on either side of this zone. Among their amenities: front-row seats to the next Big One. And fault features along the San Jacinto fault can be found near the I-10/I-215 interchange. (See chapter 6 for a more detailed discussion of the San Jacinto fault and these features.)

But as is so often the case, perhaps the best way to appreciate the faults of the Inland Empire is to stand back and view the area from either the air or a topographic map. From this perspective the faults take shape in all their glory—and in all their real and present danger.

The San Gabriel Valley

Los Angeles area newspapers might give the impression that outside of the Los Angeles Basin there is a single separate valley of any consequence: the San Fernando Valley. "The Valley" is sandwiched between the Santa Monica Mountains to the south and the Transverse Ranges to the north. I will discuss The Valley in due time, but, in an east-to-west progression, we must first look at Los Angeles' *other* valley: the San Gabriel.

For a region that might easily suffer an identity crisis, the San Gabriel Valley scarcely lacks for character. Its largest city, Pasadena, was founded in 1874, largely as a playground and health refuge for the wealthy. It has since grown into a thriving cultural and technical center. Other San Gabriel communities include Arcadia, home to the Santa Anita Race Track, and the historic town of El Monte, founded around 1850 near the end of the Santa Fe Trail.

The edges of the San Gabriel Valley are irregular, defined by several mountain ranges. The largest, the San Gabriel Mountains to the north, are part of the Transverse Ranges. The borders to the west, east, and south are more complex, formed by a series of smaller mountains including the Puente Hills to the southeast and the Verdugo Mountains to the west.

Finding faults in the San Gabriel Valley is not difficult. We can look first to its edges, where faults pass along the base of virtually every mountain that bounds the valley. In one notable case, we can also find a fault within the valley—the Raymond fault, the subtle surface manifestation that gives but little hint of the hazard it portends.

But first things first—namely, the San Gabriel Mountains themselves. At the base of these mountains is a complex and not entirely understood thrust-fault system. (I use the single term, thrust fault, throughout this book, as illustrated in chapter 2. Geologists, however, use the term only to describe faults that dip at a shallow angle. They call more steeply dipping thrust faults, such as the Sierra Madre, reverse faults.) In spite of the uncertainties, most geologists think that along most of the foothills the most active fault in this system is the Sierra Madre—the primary thrust fault along which the San Gabriels are currently being lifted. On geologic maps, the Sierra Madre fault usually shows as a series of five main fault segments that may carry separate names but are generally thought to be part of a single system.

As we saw in chapter 2, thrust—or reverse—faults can be hard to find. The Sierra Madre fault, which lies at the base of mountains that routinely experience torrential winter rains, provides a prime case in point. Along the base of the San Gabriel Mountains, we can generally find mudflows far more easily than faults. However, we can see the Sierra Madre, and other faults that make up the system, in a number of locations—locations that tend to be well visited by earth scientists and earth-science students.

To begin a fault tour of the San Gabriel Valley, we might start in the city of Arcadia and drive north to the city-owned Arcadia Wilderness Park in the foothills, where we can find a strand of the Sierra Madre fault system cutting diagonally through the face of a steep hillside. The Wilderness Park is on Highland Oaks Drive in Arcadia, just east of Santa Anita Drive. As we enter the park down a steep driveway, we can see the fault exposed in the side of the canyon facing the parking lot closest to the street. Continuing erosional forces leave the fault trace messy, but we can identify it based on the juxtaposition of rock types—a layer of older, hard rock thrust up over younger sedimentary rock. It can be a little difficult for the untrained eye to spot the fault, but finding the right part of the park is not difficult. For more guidance, ask one of the park rangers, all of whom have had plenty of experience with geologic tourists.

Heading west from Arcadia, we can drive to the northwestern edge of Pasadena, to the famed Jet Propulsion Laboratory (JPL), which has primary responsibility for unmanned space missions. Driving west on I-210 along the foothills, our course

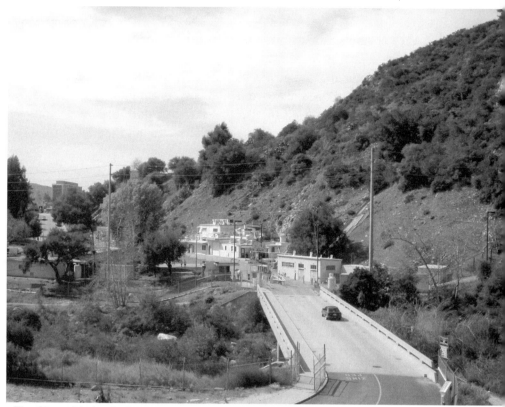

The Sierra Madre fault creates a prominent, steep scarp that cuts through the back (north) side of the Jet Propulsion Laboratory campus in Pasadena. (34 12.18N 118 9.94W)

parallels that of the Sierra Madre fault system but is offset about a mile to the south. South of the freeway along this stretch are the Verdugos, a sliver of a mountain range bounded on the south by the Verdugo fault, which runs just north of I-134. The Sierra Madre fault itself hugs the foothills north of I-210. Leaving the freeway at the JPL exit and heading north, we can find another clear and much-visited exposure of the fault near the creek beneath the abutments of JPL's east bridge. The fault scarp looms over the entire JPL campus, high and ominously steep. To the east of JPL we find residential neighborhoods—and a series of lovely homes whose spectacular views are afforded by the high and steep fault scarp.

As late as the 1990s, earth scientists debated the potential for the Sierra Madre fault to generate large earthquakes. Throughout recorded history, the greater fault system—including a number of secondary faults—has generated only fairly modest earthquakes, such as the 1990 M5.2 Upland earthquake and the 1991 M5.8 Sierra Madre earthquake. (There is, however, some debate, as we'll learn later in this chapter, about whether the 1971 San Fernando earthquake occurred on the Sierra Madre fault as well.) Were they to rupture end-to-end, each individual segment within the Sierra Madre system is large enough to generate earthquakes "only" about as large as the 1971 San Fernando and 1994 Northridge temblors, both of which were M6.7. But through the 1990s, scientists continued to find evidence that large earthquakes are able to blast through fault offsets at least as large as those seen in the Sierra Madre.

Then in 1998, geologists Charlie Rubin, Scott Lindvall, and Tom Rockwell dug a trench across the Sierra Madre fault in the town of Altadena. Geologic trenches, typically a few feet wide and dug to a depth of about 10 feet with commercial backhoes, allow geologists to observe a fault—and, they hope, to find evidence of geologic disruptions, such as fault motion, caused by past earthquakes. At this site, the fault generates a scarp that they excavated to examine the near-surface sediments. Rubin and his team found evidence for two major earthquakes. The disruption of sediments provided an estimate of the movement, or slip, in each earthquake, which in turn allowed for an estimation of the magnitude of these prehistoric earthquakes—not 6.7, but closer to 7.5. Carbon-14 dating of charcoal in the

Charlie Rubin and the Sierra Madre Fault

In the assessment of regional earthquake hazard, scientists typically face a vexing problem: how to determine the maximum size of an earthquake that can occur on a given fault or fault system. While it is often nearly impossible to say that an earthquake of a given size (within generally reasonable limits) absolutely *cannot* occur in a certain location, there is one way to show that earthquakes of a certain size can occur: to find evidence that such earthquakes occurred in the past. When Charlie Rubin and his colleagues dug a trench on the Sierra Madre fault just a stone's throw away from Pasadena, they found compelling evidence to help settle what at the time was an ongoing debate. With the myriad uncertainties that inevitably plague any analysis in the earth sciences, paleo-seismological investigations—to not only find faults but to study the past earthquakes that have occurred on them—can provide tremendously important information for hazard assessment. Such investigations have uncertainties of their own, of course, but in a very real sense they commonly represent the closest we can get—short of watching an earthquake rupture before our eyes—to ground truth.

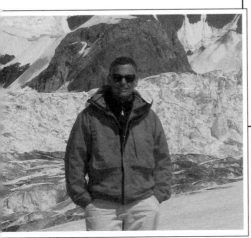

Charlie Rubin on Susitna Glacier in Alaska, where he traveled to map the surface rupture on the 2002 M7.9 Denali earthquake.
—KERRY SIEH PHOTO

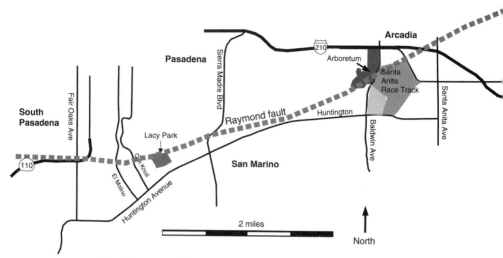

The Raymond fault cuts through the towns of Arcadia, San Marino, and South Pasadena. Along much of this trace, the fault creates a prominent scarp.

sediments revealed that the earthquakes struck between 1,100 and 15,000 years ago. The good news, then, is that such an earthquake apparently only happens once every few thousand years, so people are unlikely to experience such an event in their lifetime. The bad news is that when this earthquake does strike, it will pack a destructive wallop many times greater than that of the Northridge earthquake.

The further bad news is that the Sierra Madre fault system is scarcely the only concern for residents of the San Gabriel Valley. In 1988, the relatively modest M4.9 Pasadena earthquake called attention to another enigmatic fault in the region, the Raymond fault. The epicenter of this earthquake was right in the heart of downtown Pasadena—just a few short miles from Caltech and the Pasadena office of the U.S. Geological Survey. It would be fair to say that this temblor received more attention than most M5.0 earthquakes that shake California.

The Pasadena earthquake was far more than a rude wake-up call for local seismologists, however. It provided important new information about the Raymond fault, which had been the subject of debate for many years. This fault, which branches away from the Sierra Madre fault near Arcadia and heads westward through the communities of San Marino and South Pasadena, is associated with a modest but prominent scarp along much of its length.

Readers familiar with the Pasadena area might find themselves puzzled at this point. San Marino and South Pasadena are several miles south of the epicenter of the 1988 Pasadena earthquake, so how can this be the same fault? The answer is simple: the fault is not vertical, but rather it dips steeply toward the north, away from its surface trace. The modest 1990 temblor occurred about 10 miles (16 kilometers) below the surface and, therefore, north of the mapped surface scarp.

Showing no socioeconomic favoritism whatsoever, this fault scarp winds its way past the Los Angeles Arboretum in Arcadia and generates the small hills immediately adjacent to the San Marino Tennis Club. This particular fault is easy to find in a number of locations. Heading south from the I-210 freeway on Baldwin Avenue, the road drops abruptly at the fault scarp just before we reach the arboretum entrance on the right and the Santa Anita Mall entrance on the left. In San Marino, a more gradual bump in the road exists on Sierra Madre Boulevard just north of Huntington Drive. Farther west, the fault winds its way along the northern edge of San Marino's Lacy Park. At one time, the park was a small lake, Lake Wilson, nestled next to a small kink, or releasing bend, in the fault that creates a small zone of extension in the midst of a region of compression. At one point, Lake Wilson was dammed to provide reliable irrigation for surrounding communities, including nearby San Gabriel.

Before 1988, geologists had debated whether motion on the Raymond fault was predominantly strike-slip (lateral) or thrust. There was geologic evidence for both left-lateral and thrust motion on the fault, but left-lateral strike-slip motion seemed hard to explain given the overall compressional forces in the region.

When an earthquake occurs, though, seismologists can deduce its style of faulting from detailed analysis of the waves it generates. When researchers analyzed the data from the Pasadena earthquake, the results were unambiguous: the

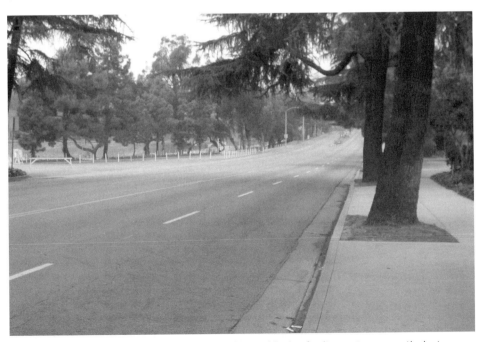

Near the Santa Anita Race Track, the Sierra Madre fault creates a gentle but pronounced scarp that cuts across Colorado Avenue and then continues along the northern side of the racetrack grounds. (34 8.70N, 118 2.47W)

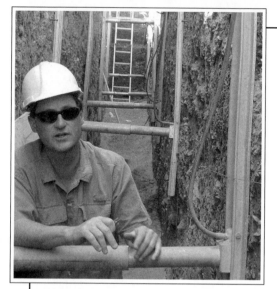

James Dolan stands in the trench he and his students excavated across the San Cayetano fault.

James Dolan, Los Angeles Fault Finder

Although USC Professor James Dolan's interests in active faulting have taken him all over the world, his interest in faults in his own backyard—the greater Los Angeles region—has never waned. With students and colleagues, James has trenched a dizzying list of faults in the area, including the Raymond, Hollywood, and San Cayetano faults. Paleoseismic investigations of trenches sometimes involve interpretation of subtle sedimentary features. But there was nothing subtle about the offset that Dolan and his students identified in a trench of the San Cayetano fault: more than 20 feet (7 meters) of slip, which they inferred to have occurred in a single earthquake. Earlier work had suggested that the fault might have ruptured in the known historic earthquake on December 21, 1812, but the documented effects of that event were much smaller than expected for a rupture with 20 feet of slip. Dolan therefore concludes that the event happened earlier, probably not long before the start of California's short historic record—one more bit of evidence that the greater Los Angeles metropolitan area is sometimes rocked by much larger earthquakes than it has seen during its short recorded history.

earthquake had produced primarily left-lateral strike-slip motion, with only a small component (about 7 percent of the total) of vertical motion.

About a decade later, geologist Dick Crook excavated the Raymond fault at the Los Angeles Arboretum and found evidence that the last surface-rupturing earthquake on this fault occurred 1,000 to 2,000 years ago. James Dolan and Kristin Weaver also excavated on the fault in San Marino, in the middle of the median strip on Sierra Madre Boulevard.

Still farther west from Sierra Madre Boulevard in San Marino, the fault creates a more prominent ridge, including the hill upon which the storied Ritz-Carlton Hotel is perched. To find this fault, simply head north on Oak Knoll Avenue from Huntington Drive until the abrupt increase in slope across the road just south of the hotel.

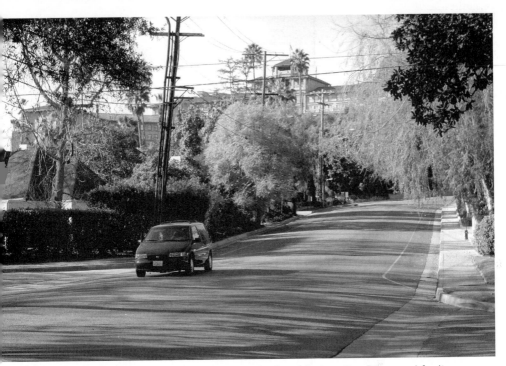

Along Oak Knoll Avenue, a residential street in San Marino, the Raymond fault creates a scarp at the base of low hills along the border between San Marino and Pasadena. The Ritz-Carlton Hotel, visible in this photo at upper left, sits at the top of the scarp.

Returning to Huntington Drive, continue 0.25 mile west to El Molino Avenue and turn north to find another good view of the fault scarp after 0.75 mile. This scarp, which runs through a lovely neighborhood, is particularly attractive in late May and early June when the blooming jacaranda trees add vibrant splashes of soft purple to the overhead tree canopy.

Retracing our steps back to Huntington Drive once again, we can continue west 1.25 miles to Fair Oaks Avenue in South Pasadena and hang a right. After driving approximately 1 mile, we reach Raymond Hill, the feature from which the fault derives its name. Development has obscured the morphology of the hill; its sharper features are now hard to recognize amid the clutter of commercial and residential real estate. Historical photographs, however, show the feature in full glory, with the Raymond Hill Hotel perched atop a steep, narrow hill that is so characteristic of fault-controlled topography. The Raymond Hill Hotel no longer exists, having given way to homes, large apartment complexes, and a few businesses.

Geologic evidence collected to date suggests that the Raymond fault is capable of producing earthquakes at least as large as M6.7. It could, however, generate much larger events, especially if it were to rupture in conjunction with another

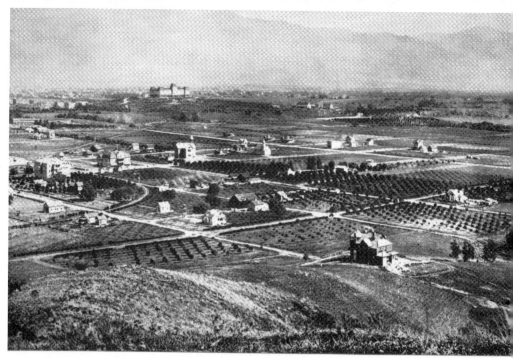

A historical photograph of the (now defunct) Raymond Hill Hotel reveals the distinct scarp that the Raymond fault created in this location *(upper left)*. The scarp, and hill, still exist, but commercial development has significantly obscured them.

fault, such as the Hollywood fault (which we'll look at later in this chapter). Once again we are left with a good news/bad news result: a fault that produces infrequent but potentially very large earthquakes.

The earthquake concerns of the San Gabriel Valley do not stop there. The strongest earthquake to shake parts of this valley in recent memory—the 1987 M6.0 Whittier earthquake—did not happen on either the Sierra Madre or the Raymond faults, but rather on the Puente Hills fault system, which is south of the valley. That fault, however, does not rightfully "belong to" the San Gabriel Valley, and so we'll discuss it in the following section. But earthquakes on that fault certainly have the potential to shake the area. When it comes to both mountains and potential earthquake sources, the San Gabriel Valley is literally surrounded—not only on all sides, but also underneath.

Like all southland valleys and basins, the San Gabriel faces significant additional hazard from the effects of amplification. When the M7.3 Landers earthquake tore through the Mojave Desert in 1992, the waves it generated were large enough to wake the dead—or at least the dead-tired—in the San Gabriel Valley. At its most severe point, shaking strong enough to knock objects off of shelves continued for at least a minute in some locations. And after the strong shaking had subsided, a gentle "sloshing" of the ground could be felt if one stood very still. These delayed reverberations—waves perhaps two to three seconds long from peak to peak—were caused by energy that was trapped within the valley sediments, producing relatively slow and prolonged ripples that seismologists call surface waves.

Although powerful, the Landers earthquake struck some distance from the San Gabriel Valley. When a big shock hits closer to home, it will also very likely generate surface waves of its own—and they are unlikely to be gentle reverberations.

"The Valley" and Points West

Driving westward from the San Gabriel Valley over the Verdugo Hills, we reach The Valley—that is, the San Fernando Valley, which stretches from Glendale to Chatsworth. The impetus for initial settlement of this large valley was, at least to some extent, less than noble. In its early years, San Fernando was the destination of choice for those embarked on "white flight" from the inner-city tumult of Los Angeles proper. In 1950, only a tiny fraction of the residents of the San Fernando Valley were ethnic minorities. Euphemistically The Valley was viewed as a "safe" (wink) place to raise one's children—one with "good" (wink) schools.

Those roots seem ironic now, for by the end of the twentieth century, the San Fernando Valley had become as diverse as the rest of the greater Los Angeles region. Yet The Valley remains a geographically and to some extent culturally distinct (think, like, Valley Girls) region. Geologically speaking, the San Fernando Valley is closely linked to the region one step farther west: the Ventura Basin. Although the Simi Hills separate the two geologic provinces, the tectonic forces at work in the Ventura Basin are closely related to those in the San Fernando Valley.

Like the San Gabriel Valley to the east, the San Fernando Valley and the Ventura Basin are bounded by mountains, in this case the Verdugos to the east, the San Gabriels to the north, and the Santa Monica Mountains to the south. And here again, finding faults generally involves looking to those mountains.

Considering only the geology and topography of the San Fernando Valley, however, faults are relatively difficult to find. The faults that ring this corner of southern California are, as a rule, complex. Much of the earthquake hazard in this region stems from the system of faults that runs along the base of the San Gabriel Mountains. This complex fault system includes individual faults that dip both to the north and to the south.

The Santa Susana thrust fault, which itself consists of numerous segments, runs approximately 23 miles (38 kilometers) westward from the town of San Fernando toward the small town of Piru. Most but not all of the fault segments dip down to the north.

The Santa Susana fault is notable among the myriad complex faults in the Los Angeles area in that it has ruptured in a large earthquake within recorded history. One short segment of this fault system apparently ruptured in 1971 in

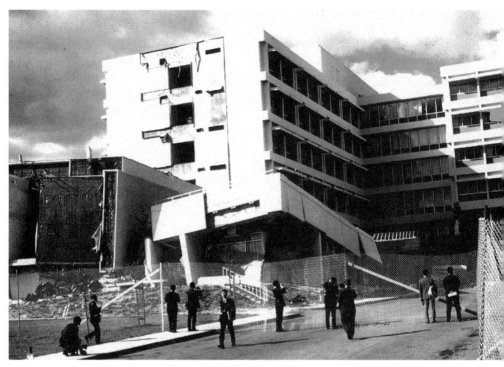

Damage to Olive View Hospital following the 1971 Sylmar (San Fernando) earthquake

the M6.7 San Fernando earthquake, bringing to an end the nearly four decades of seismic quiescence that the greater Los Angeles region had enjoyed. Geologically, the San Fernando earthquake highlights the complexity of southern California's large fault systems. Although many geologists (and the official Web site of the southern California Earthquake Center) place the earthquake on the eastern edge of the Santa Susana fault, other scientists consider the segment to be part of the Sierra Madre fault. The matter is less a real debate than an indication that the distinction between these two fault systems, and the precise location and significance of the boundary between them, is largely semantic and arguably irrelevant.

Whatever one calls its causative fault, the San Fernando earthquake, also sometimes known as the Sylmar quake, served as a dramatic reminder that southern California is earthquake country, and left in its wake a level of damage few residents of southern California had seen before.

The San Fernando earthquake still ranks among the most damaging earthquakes in California history. Its epicenter was in the mountains well north of Sylmar along I-5, but its rupture extended southwestward through Sylmar and slightly beyond. The temblor claimed fifty-eight lives and caused more than half a billion dollars in property damage (in 1971 dollars). Two area hospitals suffered

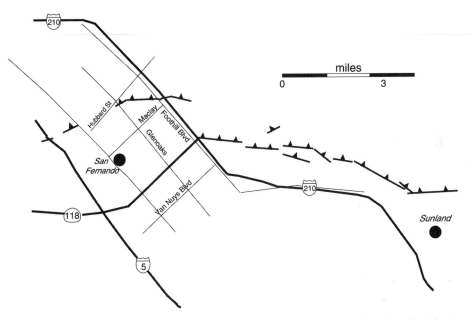

Mapped surface rupture from the 1971 San Fernando earthquake. Dark lines indicate surface faulting mapped in 1971; at depth, the thrust faults angle down in the direction of the small triangles.

major damage and revealed critical flaws in a style of building design that experts had thought provided sufficient resistance to shaking. We can see the new Olive View Hospital, rebuilt on the same site in Sylmar but with a much different design, from the northbound I-210 at the base of the mountains just north of the Roxford Street exit.

The San Fernando earthquake occurred on a fault segment that dipped steeply down to the north under the San Gabriel Mountains. The rupture did reach the surface, producing average displacements of about 3 feet (1 meter) along the fault trace. Bob Yerkes and other geologists mapped surface rupture along four distinct segments: 1) south of the Van Norman reservoir between I-5 and I-405; 2) a short Mission Wells segment about half a mile east of segment 1; 3) a Tujunga segment that runs along the base of the San Gabriel Mountains about 3 miles (5 kilometers) toward the west from Sunland; and 4) a Sylmar segment that runs about 1.2 miles (2 kilometers) through the town of Sylmar.

The most dramatic breaks were along the Sylmar segment, beginning near the intersection of Hubbard Street and Glenoaks Boulevard in Sylmar and extending eastward through the town of San Fernando, across I-210, to the San Fernando Industrial Park. Immediately after the earthquake, many geologists rushed to the mountain front to search for a scarp along what they knew from seismological data to be a thrust earthquake. Yet some of the most dramatic surface features—everything but the Tujunga segment—lie west of I-210, not along the mountains at all but well into the valley. The location of these breaks reflects the angle at which the fault dips as well as the complexity of the Santa Susana and San Gabriel thrust-fault systems. Time and the dark forces of road repair and urban development have softened these once-crisp features, but as we drive north on I-210, we can see the steepness of the mountain front near and just west of Sunland, standing in testimony to the presence of an active fault.

The Tujunga segment ran from Sunland to near the current intersection of I-210 and California 118. The rupture continued westward along the Sylmar segment, but this piece of the rupture is offset northward by a little less than a mile.

The best place to find faults in San Fernando is along the Sylmar segment. Taking the Hubbard exit off of I-210 and driving about a mile southwest, we arrive at Glenoaks Avenue. Some of the clearest surface breaks were just south of this intersection. Time has worn smooth the edges of the offset, but a small piece of it was landscaped and preserved in the parking lot of a McDonald's restaurant just below the intersection. It appears that the restaurant and parking lot were built after the earthquake, and that the owners decided to landscape the scarp rather than smooth it out (or have a pesky bump in their parking lot).

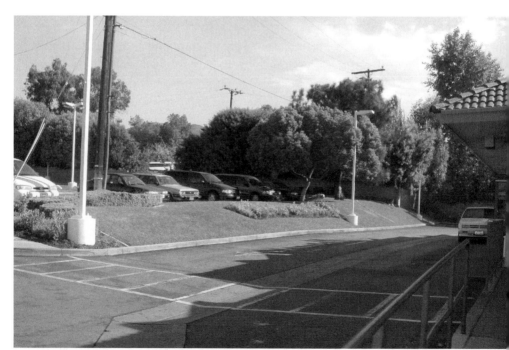

Burgers and shakes, California style. A small segment of the 1971 surface rupture runs east-west through what is now a McDonald's parking lot. (34.298N, 118.441W)

The 1971 rupture continues almost due east from here to near the intersection of Foothill Boulevard and Maclay Avenue. The roads, however, are oriented on a southwest-northeast grid, which makes finding faults something of a scavenger hunt. As we cross I-210 on Maclay, the fault is to our immediate north. Here it starts to run along the base of the hills: from this point eastward, the fault is associated with the topographic slope break typical of thrust faults. The fault has created hills that we can see from I-210 just north of the Maclay exit.

The San Fernando main shock holds an important place in the annals of modern seismology because it was among the first to be studied in detail with so-called strong motion data. Seismologists collect strong motion data using specialized instruments built to record only large earthquakes, and to record the ground motions on scale (that is, without hitting the stops). This is in contrast to most earthquake-monitoring instruments deployed earlier in the twentieth century, which were designed to be very sensitive to small ground motions, but which typically went off scale (that is, reached a point of saturation) for earthquakes greater than M3.

Researchers exploited the data from the San Fernando main shock in a couple of important ways, both to study the reverberations within the San Fernando Valley and to explore the complexity of the main-shock rupture. The latter investigations revealed the event to have been quite complicated, with some studies inferring that the rupture had involved two distinct, nearly parallel faults.

Nearly three decades after the San Fernando earthquake, scientists' attention was called back to data collected from that event—not to the strong motion data but to a perplexing observation that had been made by scientists in the field after the earthquake struck. On the sides of a road that the rupture had cut, bent pipes showed that the two sides of the fault had been squished together, a process geologists term shortening. Yet the pavement of the road, while cracked, remained mostly smooth, revealing no evidence of one side of the fault pushing up over the other. Unable to make sense of it, the scientists filed away the observation, yet another geological conundrum.

Then in the late 1990s, theoretical and observational investigations of thrust faults began to show that the ground motions of the so-called hanging wall— the side of a thrust fault that moves upward—can be extremely large. As seismologist James Brune and others argued, this effect reflects basic dynamic properties of a thrust-fault rupture. Looking back to the seemingly unperturbed road in San Fernando, seismologists made an intriguing suggestion: perhaps the ground motions were strong enough to fling up the asphalt as the fault ruptured beneath it; and once the rupture came to a stop, the road surface fell smoothly back into place over the fault scarp. The ground motions this scenario implies would have to be extremely powerful to counter the force of gravity holding down the road—not to mention the degree of adhesion binding the surface to the dirt

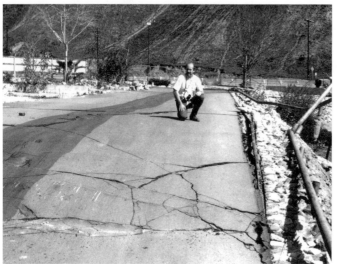

Lloyd Cluff examines the surface rupture of the 1971 San Fernando earthquake, which cut across this road. The thrust motion of the fault compressed and broke the pipe on the side of the fault, a process geologists call shortening. The pavement itself, however, revealed no evidence of compression, leading to speculation that the road surface was flung into the air as the fault moved beneath it.
—CLARENCE ALLEN PHOTO

underneath. No other tenable explanations have been advanced, which makes the theory attractive, albeit sobering.

Fortunately, much of the strongest shaking from the San Fernando earthquake took place very close to the fault, up in the mountains. This included shaking at one seismometer, near Pacoima Dam, that recorded a maximum shaking level of 1.7 times the acceleration caused by gravity—one of the strongest shaking levels ever recorded. When the earthquake struck, many seismologists and engineers had been skeptical that ground motions even as large as 100 percent of the force of gravity were possible, let alone 200 percent.

Researchers devoted many years of study to the Pacoima Dam recording. Some seismologists and engineers argued that it must have been a fluke—that the extremely rugged topography near the dam had produced such extraordinary shaking. But theoretical studies and subsequent high-amplitude records made of other large earthquakes argued that the Pacoima Dam record was not without precedent. Scary, yes, but freakish, no.

The strongest shaking from the San Fernando earthquake may have occurred in the mountains, but damage within the more densely populated valley was a testament to the level of shaking that struck there as well. Longtime residents of the San Fernando Valley may have felt that they had "their earthquake," but they would have another just a few decades later. At 4:31 A.M. on January 17, 1994, the Northridge earthquake struck, rupturing a fault segment immediately west of the 1971 rupture. Identified foreshocks did not precede this earthquake, although in the days before the temblor struck, a small sequence of M2 to M3 earthquakes shook the Santa Monica region. It remains unclear whether these small events were in any way related to the Northridge main shock. They clearly

During earthquake

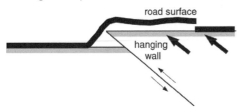

After earthquake

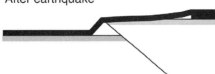

The proposed explanation for the apparent lack of compression on the road surface. Motion on the thrust fault flings the pavement into the air *(top)*, allowing it to drape smoothly over the scarp once the fault stops moving *(bottom)*. The overall width of the pavement has been reduced, or shortened, not over the fault, but to the right of the fault, where two layers of pavement overlap.

Rupture reaches surface

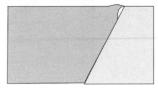

Detachment ("fling") at toe of hanging wall

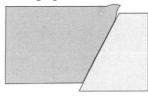

After earthquake

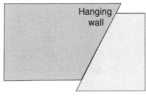

The concept of "fault fling," whereby motion along an angled thrust fault can cause extremely high ground motions at the tip of the upper, or hanging, block of crust

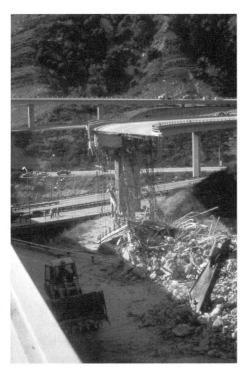

The collapse of the I-14/I-5 freeway interchange was one of the most dramatic, and potentially dangerous, consequences of the 1994 Northridge earthquake. Fortunately, the freeways were nearly empty when the earthquake struck at 4:31 A.M. local time, but a highway patrolman on a motorcycle was killed at this site.

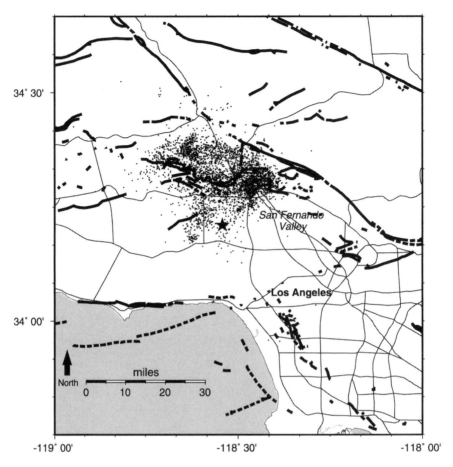

The epicenter of the January 17, 1994, Northridge earthquake *(star)*
and aftershocks recorded during the first two weeks of the sequence

were not classic foreshocks, which by definition occur only a short distance (a few miles, perhaps) from their main shock.

Whether or not the Northridge earthquake had foreshocks, the main shock itself packed a powerful punch. It claimed several dozen lives and a staggering forty billion dollars in property damage, including spectacular (and in one case, deadly) collapses of two major freeways: I-10 near La Cienega south of Northridge, and the I-5/I-14 interchange in the mountains north of the epicenter.

The magnitude of the Northridge earthquake proved to be nearly identical to that of the San Fernando earthquake, although it ruptured a south-dipping fault that runs beneath the valley. By analyzing data from the main shock and early aftershocks, seismologists determined the orientation of the fault very quickly. However, they were not able to point to a fault trace on a map and identify the specific fault that had ruptured during the earthquake. This led to considerable consternation among the media and the public about whether this damaging earthquake had occurred on a "previously unknown" fault.

Earth scientists had known full well that complex fault systems run through the San Fernando Valley, including both north- and south-dipping segments. Unquestionably, however, the Northridge temblor provided further evidence for just how complex these fault systems are.

The seismotourist hoping to find the Northridge fault is out of luck: unlike the Santa Susana fault, this fault segment is blind. Seismologists eventually determined the epicenter of the Northridge earthquake to be at the corner of Roscoe and Reseda Boulevards, very close to the border between Northridge and the neighboring town of Reseda. However, there isn't much of geologic interest to see at that intersection because the fault is about 12 miles (20 kilometers) beneath the surface.

Many geologists think that the Northridge fault should be considered part of the larger Oak Ridge fault system that extends to the west. The Oak Ridge fault proper is a south-dipping (probably non-blind) thrust fault that extends fully 56 miles (90 kilometers) through the charming towns of Santa Paula, Fillmore, and Ventura. Along much of its length, this fault is not hard to find. Its scarp is evident as a pronounced ridge that parallels California 126 between the town of Piru and the coast. The surface trace peters out as it passes eastward, leading some geologists to think that it continues toward Northridge as a blind thrust.

And therein lies the geologic link between the Ventura Basin and the San Fernando Valley. It is entirely possible that both the Oak Ridge and the Santa Susana faults do not respect the geographic boundary that separates the two regions. And it will come as no surprise by now to hear that this has important implications for earthquake hazard. The appreciable combined length of the Oak Ridge fault, upwards of 56 miles (90 kilometers), implies that it can potentially rupture in very large earthquakes.

Concern for earthquake hazard in the Ventura Basin specifically had been raised very shortly before the Northridge main shock struck. Looking at recent data from Global Positioning System (GPS) satellites, geophysicist Andrea Donnellan led a team that confirmed earlier suggestions that the Ventura Basin was undergoing unusually high rates of compression, or squeezing. If substantial energy, or strain, is building on a fault, then detailed GPS measurements can reveal the location of possible fault rupture because such data can track the ground warping associated with building strain. Rarely is science as well timed as it was in Donnellan's case, in which observations of strain buildup preceded an earthquake by only a few short years.

Some questions remain about the earthquake "forecast" that resulted from Donnellan's study, as that analysis revealed a strain buildup farther west than

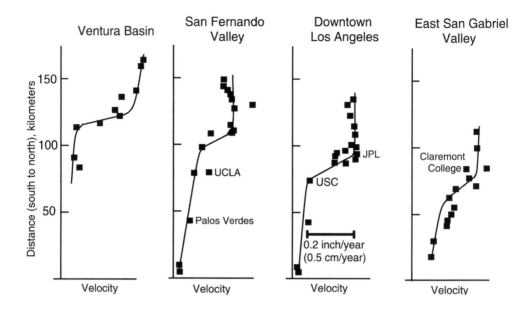

Data collected from GPS instruments reveal how deformation, or strain, is building in the Ventura region and other regions throughout southern California. Individual data points in each panel correspond to estimates of ground velocity. The kinks in these values along each profile, as highlighted by the smooth lines, indicate zones where the velocity of the ground is changing over a relatively short distance; these correspond to the regions where strain is accumulating, presumably along faults. (Velocity scale is the same in all four panels.) —FROM WORK BY DON ARGUS AND OTHERS

the Northridge region. For this and other reasons, residents of the San Fernando Valley and Ventura Basin should know that, even after two major temblors they would be ill-advised to be sanguine about earthquake hazard.

To continue on a tour of faults farther west from the San Fernando Valley, we can drive north on I-5 to California 126 and head west along a small valley that widens into the Ventura Basin. This valley is currently being squeezed, the valley floor moving downward relative to the mountains on both sides. The motion occurs along two fault systems, a south-dipping fault on the south side of the valley and a north-dipping fault on the north side.

The fault that defines the northern edge of the Ventura Basin, the San Cayetano, has been the subject of detailed paleoseismic investigations in recent years. James Dolan and his students have excavated two trenches just north of the small community of Piru and found dramatic evidence for at least one large, surface-rupturing event within the last 350 years. The date of the most recent event, obtained from carbon-14 dating, is consistent with the date of a known historical earthquake in California: a December 21, 1812, temblor that damaged missions

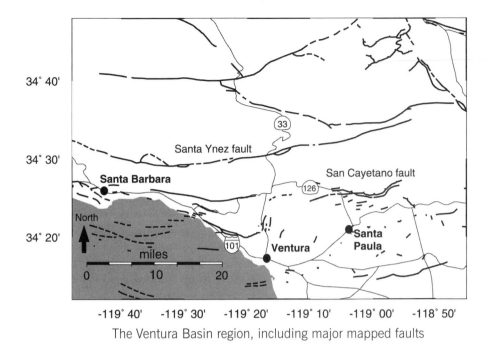

The Ventura Basin region, including major mapped faults

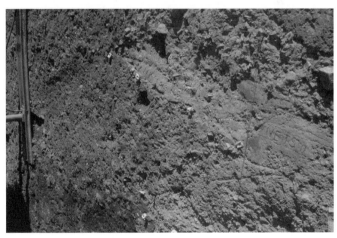

this trench that James lan and his students 'estigated, an offset layer of ung sedimentary rock (the ,ooth, light band in the per center, slanting down the right) provides clear dence of substantial)vement along the San yetano fault. In this photo, : fault trace runs down gonally to the left from the ge of the sediment wedge.

in Ventura and Santa Barbara. However, trench investigations in 2002 revealed compelling evidence for substantial surface slip, perhaps as much as 20 to 26 feet (6 to 8 meters)—a major temblor, probably too large to be consistent with the level of damage that the 1812 temblor caused. It appears, then, that the last large earthquake on the San Cayetano fault probably happened just prior to the start of the historic record, perhaps in the 1700s. Whenever it occurred, the event must have been impressive, producing surface slip apparently comparable to the 1999 M7.6 Chi-Chi earthquake in Taiwan.

Results of investigations of the San Cayetano fault thus served to highlight a growing consensus in the earth-science community: that earthquakes well upwards of M7.0 have shaken the greater Los Angeles Basin and almost certainly will do so again. And in the aftermath of the 1971 and 1994 earthquakes, we cannot help but wonder if there are any dominoes left to fall—that is, faults with significant stored strain that the recent earthquakes might have nudged closer to failure. The short answer is that we don't know what lies ahead. However, analysis of recent GPS data clearly shows that substantial strain is building up in the Ventura Basin region. Somewhere, sometime, it will have to be released.

The Los Angeles Basin and San Diego

Discussing southern California's regions in turn, we become aware of a repeating theme: mountains define valleys and basins, and faults create mountains. The Los Angeles Basin itself is no exception, except that along one edge it ends not at a mountain but at the coast. Unfortunately, this does little to lessen the earthquake hazard within the basin, since, as we'll see in more detail later in this chapter, faults run roughly northwest-southeast both on land along the coast and offshore. Here again, where earthquake hazard in greater Los Angeles is concerned, there is no place to hide.

There should never have been a shred of doubt about earthquake hazard in Los Angeles, because the first documented earthquakes in California occurred in this region during the first overland European expedition through the state. The first temblor struck on July 28, 1769, while Gaspar de Portolá and his expedition camped along a river about 30 miles (50 kilometers) south of present-day Los Angeles. The expedition felt a smattering of smaller earthquakes on subsequent days. Inspired by the perceived threat posed by Russian and British expansion into the north and northwest Pacific, Portolá's expedition marked the beginning of Spain's efforts to establish missions and colonize the state.

The state's welcome was less than warm. The description of shaking suggests a magnitude in the neighborhood of 6.0, and the diary of one expedition member, Father Juan Crespi, tells of at least a dozen aftershocks, some of them quite strong. The Portolá expedition, understandably, named the river Rio de los Temblores. Father Juan Crespi, who chronicled the Portolá expedition, named the place Jesus de los Temblores. But soldiers—perhaps by way of appeal—instead adopted the saint's name by which we know the river and region today: Santa Ana.

The expedition felt no aftershocks once the party was as far north as the San Fernando Valley. Because aftershocks cluster close to their main shock, the evidence suggests (albeit with major uncertainties) an epicenter somewhere in the Los Angeles Basin, possibly toward its southern end.

From the time of this inhospitable welcome, awareness of earthquake hazard and faults in the Los Angeles area developed slowly but surely, all the way up to the 1990s and early twenty-first century, during which earth scientists' understanding of faults here has grown tremendously. Historically, finding faults in this area has been difficult because the surface manifestations tend to be subtle. Two of the faults now considered among the most dangerous for Los Angeles are blind thrust faults whose existence researchers did not recognize just a few short decades ago. We'll investigate these faults—and the ingenious studies that have elucidated their properties—shortly.

But let me begin this section by discussing one LA-area fault that was not hard to find: the Newport-Inglewood. The surface expression of this fault is not particularly dramatic. It more-or-less parallels the coast, veering northwestward from Long Beach up through Beverly Hills. The fault crosses the Santa Monica Freeway (also known as the dreaded I-10) between the Robertson and La Cienega exits, but there is not much to see. Sediments carried down the mountains by the Los Angeles River are constantly obscuring the surface trace of the fault. Sedimentation and/or erosion combine to obscure the surface trace of the fault in other areas as well.

Worse yet, this is another fault that is broken into a number of distinct fault segments. In a few places, such as the southwest edge of Signal Hill, those fault segments define visible, steep, linear slopes. For the most part, however, the Newport-Inglewood fault does not cut a conspicuous swath through the region.

However, the fault was not hard to find because it called attention to itself quite early—when the M6.4 Long Beach earthquake struck on the evening of March 10, 1933. Although earthquakes this large commonly rupture faults all the way to the surface, this one did not. It was, however, large enough to exact a steep toll: 120 deaths and heavy damage to unreinforced masonry buildings. The heavily damaged or destroyed buildings included many schools, which were mercifully empty when the earthquake struck. However, the damage (and the realization that it could have been much worse) led directly to passage of the Field Act, which gave the state authority to approve the design and supervise the construction of public schools.

An energetic sequence of aftershocks followed the Long Beach earthquake, lasting for many months. Virtually all earthquakes of its size will be followed by a number of subsequent events large enough to be felt—and a larger number of even smaller events. The largest aftershock generated by an average main shock is approximately one magnitude unit smaller than its parent. But aftershock sequences vary considerably from main shock to main shock, and the one following the Long Beach earthquake was impressive indeed.

In the words of then-Long Beach resident Anne Aardema, "Quake after quake followed, about three hours lapsing between them. Some of these quakes were very severe, and did lots more damage." Miss Aardema went on to write, "In front of our house was a vacant space for a few miles. It was strange and magnificent to watch this field during a quake. It actually rolled like thousands of waves would, ripple after ripple of earth rolling and swaying." Showing herself to be a true southern Californian at heart, she concluded, "The first three or four nights, my bed had a grand time, rolling from one wall to the other during those quakes. And, there was no charge for that ride." This account of innumerous aftershocks is borne out by data. By 1933, seismologists at the California Institute of Seismology were operating seismometers that allowed rough estimates of the locations and magnitudes of the aftershocks.

Miss Aardema's account of visible ripples in a field, however, is more enigmatic. Countless observers of countless earthquakes, many of whom appear to be entirely sober and credible, have recorded similar accounts of large-amplitude waves. However, seismometers have yet to record waves that would generate the kinds of high-amplitude waves that people describe. The observations, therefore, remain a puzzle. It is possible that the ground moves in ways that scientists do not currently understand, but some scientists have suggested that the accounts result from an optical illusion related to human visual perception during strong ground motion. Either way, accounts such as Miss Aardema's provide sobering testimony to the destructive power of the Long Beach earthquake—an event that, in the larger scheme of things, was relatively modest in size.

Although the Long Beach earthquake made it clear that southern California was Earthquake Country, the greater Los Angeles region entered a remarkably quiet stretch not long afterwards. Between 1940 and 1971, when much of the region was developed, not a single earthquake of M4.5 or greater occurred there. As we already know, the 1971 San Fernando earthquake shattered the silence, and it was broken repeatedly through the late 1980s by a series of earthquakes in different locations. A couple of those earthquakes occurred in the San Gabriel Valley region and have already been discussed. The largest and most destructive to strike the San Gabriel Valley, however, was the M6.0 Whittier earthquake of 1987. This temblor caused $358 million in property damage, inflicting heavy damage on older masonry buildings in the communities of Whittier and Alhambra. Away from those regions, most single-family homes sustained relatively little damage, although many chimneys collapsed, in some cases falling through roofs.

The Whittier earthquake occurred on a fault that seismologists had not recognized before 1987. Subsequent analysis by Bob Yeats and others revealed it to be a blind thrust fault that trended roughly northwest-southeast approximately 12 miles (20 kilometers) east of downtown Los Angeles. Scientists linked that fault to ongoing uplift of the Puente Hills, and dubbed it the Elysian Park fault.

In a sobering but nifty bit of science, geologist John Shaw teamed up with seismologist Peter Shearer in the late 1990s to combine results from high-resolution earthquake location studies with geologic information gleaned from

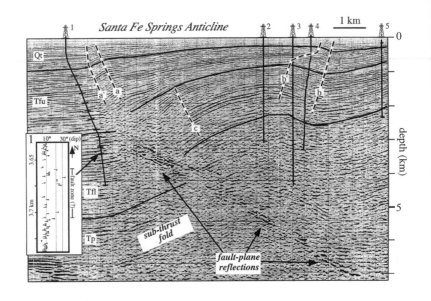

Santa Fe Springs Anticline

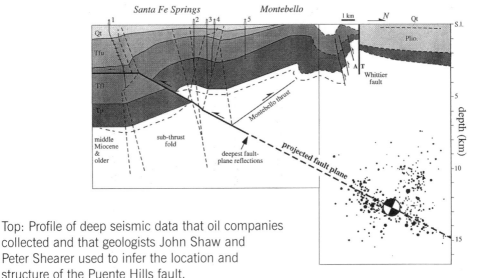

Top: Profile of deep seismic data that oil companies collected and that geologists John Shaw and Peter Shearer used to infer the location and structure of the Puente Hills fault.

Bottom: Combining the fault structure inferred from the oil companies' data with precise locations for the 1987 Whittier earthquake and its aftershocks, the structure of the Puente Hills fault came into view as shown. —FROM WORK BY JOHN SHAW AND PETER SHEARER

oil companies. This study succeeded in identifying a different blind thrust fault than researchers had previously proposed—one that caused the 1987 temblor and was large enough to produce far bigger earthquakes. Shaw and Shearer identified three distinct segments of this fault, which could produce earthquakes as large

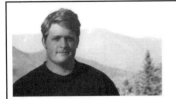

John Shaw
—COURTESY
JOHN SHAW

Men in Black

Harvard geologist John Shaw has had great success finding faults, not by scratching around the surface of the earth but by analyzing the wiggles created by small explosions. These techniques, first developed for oil exploration, rely on small explosions to generate seismic waves that travel into the earth and reflect back, typically at boundaries between softer and harder layers of rock. Because controlled explosions create the energy source, specially deployed seismometers can record them well. Both the oil industry and earth scientists now employ these so-called reflection seismology techniques. Where oil industry data are available, they can represent a boon to scientists because such data are often prohibitively expensive to collect.

In the 1990s, Shaw obtained oil company data to test his models for how blind faults develop. With Peter Shearer, from Scripps

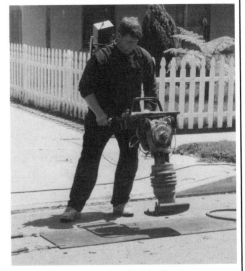

John Shaw uses a handheld reflection seismology device in a small-scale experiment. —COURTESY JOHN SHAW

Institution of Oceanography, he succeeded in imaging the complex structure of the Puente Hills fault system. The segments of this fault do not reach the surface, but their angled surfaces underlie and pose a substantial hazard to much of the northern Los Angeles Basin. And if finding faults at the surface is challenging, finding faults at depth—and figuring out how structures fit together—is a bit like studying surface geology blindfolded.

as M7.0, and named it the Puente Hills fault. The extent to which a distinct Elysian Park fault also exists in the same area remains unclear.

Because it is blind, the Puente Hills fault is not particularly spectacular at the surface. It underlies the east-trending Puente Hills, however—scarcely a small geographical feature. The Puente Hills are aligned east-west and run just south of California 60. On a street map, they are conspicuous because they lack a dense grid of surface streets, their topography having interrupted the orderly development of the valleys north and south of the hills. The fault also continues west-northwestward from the Whittier region to a well-known Los Angeles landmark: Dodger Stadium. Although buried, the angled fault lurks beneath and menaces some of the most densely populated real estate in southern California.

Just a year or two after geologists Shaw and Shearer identified the Puente Hills fault, another team of geologists identified yet another significant blind thrust fault in the Los Angeles region. In this case, geologist Lisa Grant led a group of scientists who studied elevated terraces, or "bathtub rings," that indicated ancient beaches in the Back Bay region of Newport Beach and in Crystal Cove. Grant realized that these elevated beaches suggested a long history of earthquake activity on a fault beneath the San Joaquin Hills. Using rare, tiny corals that grow in the

Lisa Grant: Finding Fault in Orange County

As a child growing up in southern California, Lisa Grant remembers looking out over the coastline and wondering why the land didn't slope down gradually to meet the ocean, but rather dropped in abrupt stair steps. As a graduate student at Caltech years later, Grant learned how faults below the earth's surface can form such steps, called marine terraces. One day she found herself looking at the coast in Orange County and recognizing a familiar landscape. At the time, there were no known active faults that could account for the marine terraces Grant was looking at, but she was motivated to launch an investigation.

Her work suggested that a major blind thrust fault underlies the San Joaquin Hills, which Grant named the San Joaquin Hills fault, along the southern margin of the southern Los Angeles Basin. By dating corals in an elevated marsh along the coast, Grant found evidence for significant coastal uplift between A.D. 1635 and 1797. Interestingly, the first account of an earthquake in California was during

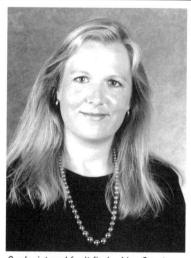

Geologist and fault finder Lisa Grant
—COURTESY LISA GRANT

this interval, written by the Gaspar de Portolá expedition in 1769. If the uplift Grant identified occurred in a single earthquake, the temblor was probably at least M7.1—probably bigger than the earthquake Portolá described. In any case, the fault clearly represents an important component of hazard in the rapidly growing Orange County region. And in the midst of the well-studied greater Los Angeles Basin, it was no small feat to discover a brand new—or rather, old but previously unknown—fault.

cold coastal waters of California to date the age of the terraces, Grant was able to estimate the long-term uplift of the hills and, therefore, the rate of motion on the fault. The fault is moving relatively slowly, perhaps three-quarters of a millimeter (about the thickness of a human fingernail) per year. But that rate, coupled with the size of the San Joaquin Hills fault, is enough to generate earthquakes as large as M7.1 about once every 2,500 years.

Once again, this fault is not easy to find—if it were, someone would have identified it long before Grant's ingenious study. Like the Puente Hills fault, however, its zone of uplift is not hard to spot. The fault itself runs roughly between I-405 and the ocean from Huntington Beach to the intersection of the I-405 and the I-5 freeways (known to LA commuters as the El Toro Y). From there the fault continues south under the San Joaquin Hills to Dana Point.

Although we can't directly observe the San Joaquin Hills fault at the surface, observations from the surface yielded clues about the history of earthquakes on this fault. From their observations that a region of coastal marsh deposits was lifted 3 to 12 feet (1 to 3.6 meters) above the current shoreline, Lisa Grant and her colleagues concluded that a earthquake of at least 7.1 ruptured the blind San Joaquin Hills thrust fault between 1635 and 1855. Further evidence suggests that the event occurred prior to the local introduction of European pollens in 1769.

Most intriguingly, Grant observed that the range of 1635–1769 includes the date of the first documented earthquake in California, the largest temblor that the Portolá expedition experienced on July 28, 1769.

We may never know for certain whether the San Joaquin Hills fault was responsible for Portolá's earthquake; some scientists conclude that Portolá's account is consistent with an earthquake of only moderate size. But there is no question that a large earthquake struck during the expedition that established the first permanent Spanish settlement in the territory that would become California. Oddly enough, this is not the only time that early European forays into North America were greeted with something other than hospitality from the earth. The great 1811–1812 New Madrid earthquakes—three temblors with magnitudes upwards of 7.0, centered in the boot-heel region of Missouri—struck a few years after the Louisiana Purchase. One of the primary New Madrid main shocks disrupted the voyage of the very first steamboat (the *New Orleans*) to travel down the Mississippi River.

Without further ruminations on coincidences, let's return to the subject at hand: faults in the Los Angeles Basin. We've discussed the three major faults running through the basin (the Newport-Inglewood and San Joaquin Hills) and along its eastern edge (the Puente Hills), but a fault tour of Los Angeles scarcely ends with just those three. A series of offshore faults runs roughly parallel to the Newport-Inglewood to the west of that fault. One of those, the Palos Verdes

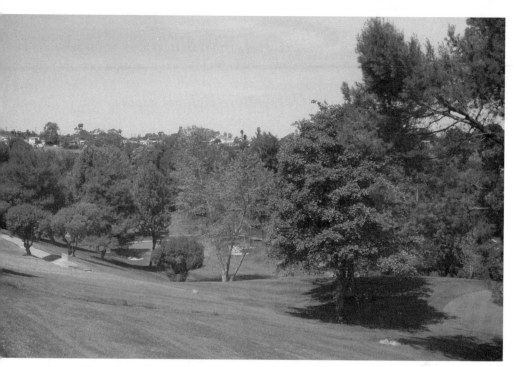

A beautifully landscaped Palos Verdes fault zone runs along a golf course. (33 46.83'N, 118 19.68'W)

fault, earns its name by cutting through the Palos Verdes peninsula. Earth scientists poorly understand the hazard associated with offshore faults, in part because they have generated no large earthquakes during recorded history, and in part because they are, well, underwater and therefore particularly tough to study. They may well represent a significant hazard for the Los Angeles region, and for the San Diego area as well.

Relative to other areas in southern California, San Diego appears fairly quiet seismologically speaking. It is far enough south and west to not feel the effects of the Big Bend in the San Andreas to the extent that the Los Angeles region does. Seismologists consider San Diego's earthquake hazard to be significantly lower than that of Los Angeles. Lower, however, does not mean zero.

Idyllic as it may seem, San Diego also has its faults. Perhaps the most studied is the Rose Canyon fault, another complex fault system that may include segments running north-northwest from San Diego Bay through La Jolla and then farther northward offshore (where it eventually connects to the Newport-Inglewood fault). Geologic investigations by Tom Rockwell and his colleagues suggest that a large earthquake created a surface rupture on the Rose Canyon fault within 125 years of A.D. 1650. Geologists have also found evidence for an earthquake to the south during this interval, in downtown San Diego.

In 2002, Lisa Grant and Tom Rockwell connected their respective dots and concluded that a zone of coastal faults stretching from the coast of Baja California north through Los Angeles had produced a series of large earthquakes between about A.D. 1640 and 1769. Geologic evidence suggests that these events followed a south-to-north progression in time. Pointing to previous suggestions that the Rose Canyon fault might connect with the Newport-Inglewood fault in Los Angeles, they further observed that the 1933 Long Beach earthquake could represent part of a northward-propagating sequence: successive major earthquakes following like dominoes over a couple of centuries. Geologists have observed a similar sequence of events on the North Anatolian fault in Turkey in recent times. If the coastal faults have experienced a migrating sequence of earthquakes in recent centuries, Grant and Rockwell observe that the next domino in line is a worrisome one: the northern Newport-Inglewood fault, which runs through the heart of the densely populated Los Angeles Basin.

But the fault map and hazard in southern California are more complex still. Another offshore San Diego fault, the Coronado Bank fault, may link up to another Los Angeles fault, the Palos Verdes. The Rose Canyon and Coronado Bay faults are two of several faults that trend in a north-northwesterly direction along California's southern coast and offshore region. Stepping eastward from the Rose Canyon fault, we find another important fault in this group: the Elsinore fault, which runs roughly along I-15 through communities such as Temecula.

In the aftermath of the devastating 1995 Kobe, Japan, earthquake, some American seismologists argued that the Kobe region could perhaps be considered an analog for the San Diego area—a region where earthquakes are not as likely as other areas, but where large and damaging events can still strike.

In 1986, at least one of San Diego's offshore faults stirred to life, producing the M5.1 Oceanside earthquake—whose shaking was felt widely. The most notable aspect of this earthquake, however, was the intense sequence of aftershocks that followed it. They numbered into the thousands and spread into a fuzzy cloud too wide to be explained by activity on a single fault. This sequence still remains enigmatic, highlighting the challenges that scientists face when they seek to study faults in the ocean. Among other issues, locating offshore earthquakes is difficult because they are recorded almost exclusively by onshore seismometers. To obtain accurate earthquake locations, recording stations must surround them.

One experiment designed to further investigate offshore faults began in 2001. It involved the deployment of underwater seismometers that will sit on the ocean floor and record small, or micro, earthquakes along the offshore faults. Such earthquakes would be too small for seismic stations on land to detect, let alone to locate with any precision. Ocean-bottom seismometers are expensive and extremely difficult to deploy and maintain, but sometimes we must go to such lengths to find faults.

Returning to land in the Los Angeles region, two additional fault systems remain in this part of our geologic tour: the Santa Monica fault system and the Hollywood fault. Both faults trend roughly east-west across the northern edge of the Los Angeles Basin.

Some geologists now think the Hollywood fault is a westward extension of the Raymond fault. Its mapped length is approximately 9 miles (15 kilometers), and it runs from the communities of Glendale westward through Beverly Hills and Hollywood itself. It has not generated a large earthquake in recorded history, but geologists think it accommodates both strike-slip (left-lateral) and thrust motion—predominantly strike slip.

If the fault ruptures by itself, its size and overall slip rate are sufficient to generate a Pretty Big One—M5.8 to M6.5—perhaps every 1,600 years. However, if the fault is a continuation of the Raymond fault, which is itself 16 miles (26 kilometers) long, then the combined faults could generate a much larger earthquake, perhaps even greater than M7.0. Once again, we would expect earthquakes of this magnitude only infrequently, on the order of every 3,000 to 5,000 years.

The Hollywood fault, therefore, poses a significant hazard and concern to the densely populated Los Angeles Basin, particularly its northern edge. However, when it comes to finding fault, the Hollywood fault is (of course!) more fun than

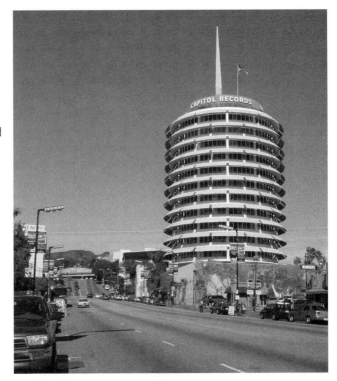

Looking north from the famed corner of Hollywood and Vine Avenues in Hollywood, the Hollywood fault creates a prominent scarp that runs east-west, just below the Capitol Records Building. (34 06.11N 118 19.59W)

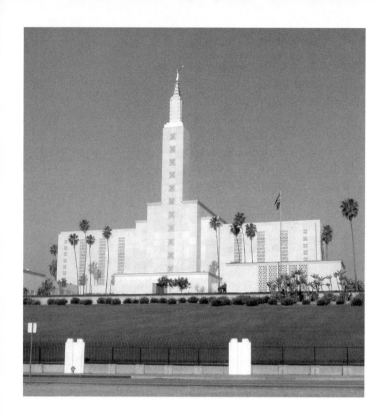

The Hollywood fault creates a prominent scarp across the lawn of the Mormon Temple, just south of the UCLA campus in Westwood. (34 3.12N 118 25.91W)

most. If we drive to the heart of Hollywood and find a parking place (good luck), we have only to walk to the famed corner of Hollywood and Vine and look northward. On the right, we will see one of Hollywood's storied landmarks, the Capitol Records Building. Looking down from this building to the street, we will find an abrupt, short hill, which is the scarp of the Hollywood fault. Past earthquakes on the fault pushed the northern side of the fault upward over the southern side. If the hill looks modest, recall that the fault moves both laterally and vertically when it ruptures.

Roughly parallel to the Hollywood fault one finds the Santa Monica fault, which, as it name suggests, is at the base of the Santa Monica Mountains and dips northward beneath them. The fault is not named for the mountains; rather, both are named after the city, whose name dates back to land grants circa 1840. This fault passes through the communities of Beverly Hills, Santa Monica, Westwood, and Pacific Palisades.

Scientists think the Santa Monica fault, like the Hollywood fault, accommodates a mix of thrust and left-lateral motion. And also like the Hollywood fault, it is not hard to find. In the west-side communities of Westwood and Brentwood, the fault generates prominent scarps that are viewable in a number of locations, including on the carefully manicured lawns of the Mormon Temple and the

Westwood Veterans hospital, and along the northern edge of the Riviera Country Club golf course.

We can reach one of the best places to find the Santa Monica fault by taking the Santa Monica exit eastward away from I-405. Approximately a mile from the freeway, we arrive at the Los Angeles Mormon Temple, the grand front lawn of which is a fault scarp—one that James Dolan has dubbed the "best landscaped fault scarp in the world."

Returning along Santa Monica Boulevard toward I-405, we can see a similar—albeit far less manicured—scarp if we look northward along many of the residential side streets. In this region, the fault scarp is within spitting distance of not only a cluster of modern high-rise buildings on Wilshire Boulevard to the north but also the UCLA campus immediately north of Wilshire.

The Santa Monica fault has not generated a large earthquake in recorded history. Much remains unknown about this fault, including a precise estimate of its slip rate and the interval between major earthquakes. From its length and overall dimensions, however, we can estimate numbers that are by now familiar: the fault appears capable of generating earthquakes as large as M7.0 approximately every few thousand years.

Interestingly, the Santa Monica fault received intense scrutiny in the 1990s not because of the earthquakes it could produce but because of the role it seems to have played in another earthquake—the 1994 Northridge temblor. Damage from this earthquake was heavy not only in the immediate vicinity of the rupture but also in the city of Santa Monica, which lies well south of Northridge.

Scientists first thought the damage in Santa Monica was caused by amplification effects related to the sediments underlying the city. But subsequent detailed

This cartoon illustrates the hypothesis that subsurface structure in the crust was responsible for a focusing effect that produced unusually high levels of shaking in Santa Monica during the 1994 Northridge earthquake.

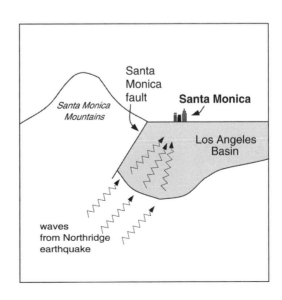

investigations by then-UCLA graduate student Xiang Gao and his colleagues suggested something more intriguing—that the dipping Santa Monica fault had formed a lens structure that had focused waves upward, with the city of Santa Monica as a focal point.

The lens theory remains controversial. Among other issues, it is clear that local sediments played some role in exacerbating the shaking. However, Gao and his colleagues presented compelling evidence for a focusing effect: the underground structure caused earthquake waves to bend in a way that amplified the shaking in Santa Monica, in the same way that a microscope can focus light waves to a single spot. Recordings of aftershocks showed that shaking in Santa Monica was unusually high only for aftershocks whose locations were close to that of the Northridge main shock. Aftershocks centered either west or east of the main shock did not generate unusual shaking patterns in Santa Monica.

Although we might—and scientists do—argue about the detailed interpretation of the Santa Monica data, the results highlight one important and unambiguous reality: when earthquakes strike anywhere in the greater Los Angeles region, their waves spread outward from the source and respond in complicated ways to the complex three-dimensional geologic structure they encounter. This structure includes basins and valleys, shallow stream deposits, and numerous faults. It is, therefore, not only possible but likely that shaking patterns from future earthquakes will be as mercurial as that generated by Northridge—and as hard to predict.

This is an important lesson to consider as we discuss specific faults in different parts of Los Angeles. Although communities immediately adjacent to each fault are at obvious risk from earthquakes on those faults, the greater Los Angeles region is not all that big. Earthquakes in one part of the region can easily affect other areas, especially within other basins and valleys where amplification effects are certain to occur. This type of influence during historic times has been relatively modest because the earthquakes themselves—Long Beach, San Fernando, Northridge—have been modest. Eventually, however, one of the major fault systems will rupture to produce an earthquake of M7.0 to M7.5. When that happens, the reverberations will echo far more loudly across the region as a whole.

Nowhere is this concern greater than within the densely populated Los Angeles Basin itself. Recent studies have shown that the great depth of the basin will make the sediment amplification effects here substantial; the effects will be even worse along the coast and some ancient stream channels where especially soft sediments exist near the surface. The basin is, moreover, ringed not only by faults but also by outlying regions with faults of their own. In Los Angeles, it is both a feel-good slogan and a geologic reality to say that "we are all in this together."

Putting the Pieces Together

All the faults we've explored in this chapter unite to contribute to the greater Los Angeles region's appreciable earthquake hazard. Earthquake hazard assessment involves, literally, adding up the potential hazard posed by each fault that stands to affect a region. This, in turn, involves assessment of the magnitudes of the largest earthquakes expected on each fault.

Looking at the faults and fault systems throughout the greater Los Angeles region, the bottom line threatens to become repetitious. According to the best available evidence, the region's major fault systems all have the potential to produce M7.0 to 7.5 earthquakes perhaps every 2,000 to 5,000 years.

Recall that earthquakes on faults such as the Sierra Madre are driven by the overall compression, or contraction, across the Los Angeles area. Researchers can estimate the amplitude of this compression both from geologic studies of faults and from studies that use GPS data to directly measure gradual crustal motion. Scientists can then use these results to predict the overall rate of earthquakes on faults in the greater Los Angeles region. This type of analysis has corroborated the conclusions based on geologic data alone.

Rupture on any one of the major faults is, therefore, unlikely to occur in any one human lifetime, or even within the lifetime of several successive generations. Unfortunately, the collective hazard is rather less benign. If each of six to eight major fault systems produces a major earthquake (not Northridge-sized, but much larger) every few thousand years, then we should expect one such earthquake, somewhere, perhaps every few hundred years—from a human perspective, a far less comforting number. Less comforting still is the growing consensus that large earthquakes tend to occur in clusters of decades to perhaps a few hundred years. The greater Los Angeles Basin has been fairly quiet throughout the short historic record; the future could be very different.

In terms of overall geology and tectonics, the faults in the Los Angeles area are, to some extent, not hard to understand considering the compression—call it the Big Squeeze—resulting from the large-scale plate-tectonic forces that give rise to the Big Bend. Squeezing the crust creates thrust faults along which vertical motion causes the crust to thicken. Simple cartoon illustrations reveal how this builds mountains over time.

But not all the faults in Los Angeles are thrust faults. The set of onshore and offshore north-northwesterly trending faults through Los Angeles and San Diego are primarily strike-slip faults. Each of these faults moves relatively slowly, and likely accommodates a small fraction of the plate boundary. The plate boundary is far wider than the San Andreas fault: the two plates do not slide past one another cleanly but instead create a zone over which California is being sliced into ribbons.

In addition to faults that, like the San Andreas, experience right-lateral strike-slip motion, both the Hollywood and Raymond faults appear to accommodate significant lateral motion, but in a left-lateral sense. In the late 1990s, Tom Rockwell and his colleagues sized up Los Angeles faults and made the intriguing suggestion that, at least to some extent, Los Angeles is characterized by "escape tectonics." Resisting the temptation to make jokes (any residents of Oregon and Washington reading this book are, of course, free to do otherwise), escape tectonics was the name Rockwell used for something that researchers had observed before in other areas and had known by other monikers, including "watermelon seed tectonics," which provides a good springboard from which to introduce the concept.

Squeeze a watermelon seed between your fingers and what happens? It doesn't compress but rather squirts sideways. Although rocks are not as slippery as watermelon seeds, blocks of crust might well be forced sideways if a region is under compression. Depending on the forces that push back when the blocks try to "escape," these blocks may be able to accommodate some of the compression with lateral motion. (As a purely disgusting aside, this is known in some [typically British] circles as "hedgehog tectonics," because when an automobile runs over a hedgehog . . . well . . . you get the idea.)

The extent to which Los Angeles is like a hedgehog remains open to debate. As intriguing as the analogy may be, it is clear that in many respects the greater Los Angeles region represents a microcosm for the state as a whole, with myriad faults defining puzzle pieces that fit together and affect one another in extraordinarily complex ways. Furthermore, the geologic diversity of this amazing region does not only parallel its cultural and socioeconomic diversity; to a very large extent the former has helped create the latter. Los Angeles' faults might be a little hard to tolerate at times. Clearly they represent a direct imperative to residents of southern California to remember the lessons of the Portolá expedition. Still, Los Angeles would not be Los Angeles—for worse but also for better—without its diverse and intricately complicated faults.

4 Finding Fault in the San Francisco Bay Area

As the nineteenth century drew to a close, Americans were well familiar with earthquakes. The city of Charleston, South Carolina, had been hard hit by an 1886 temblor now estimated to have had a magnitude of approximately 7.0. Earlier in the century, but not yet faded from memory, the 1811–1812 New Madrid sequence had rattled the boot-heel region of Missouri, producing three powerful earthquakes with magnitudes upwards (possibly well upwards) of 7.0. Because earthquake waves travel efficiently in the old, relatively unfractured crust of central and eastern North America, all of these shocks had an enormous reach. They were felt widely throughout the eastern half of the country and caused light damage at distances up to 1,000 miles (1,500 kilometers)—roughly the distance separating Los Angeles and Seattle. Imagine an earthquake in one of those western cities damaging buildings in the other!

By virtue of these eastern/central earthquakes as well as California's short historic record, as the nineteenth century drew to a close, the Golden State was known for its gold more than for its earthquakes. In his 1872 book, *The Golden State: A History of the Region West of the Rocky Mountains,* Rolander Guy McClellan discussed the New Madrid earthquakes en route to an observation that "indeed, compared with the earthquakes of other times and countries, California's earthquakes are but gentle oscillations."

We might wonder about the sobriety of a person who would make this observation while having full knowledge of the portentous earthquakes that struck the Bay Area in 1868 and the Owens Valley in 1872. However, to an early naturalist-historian with no understanding of earthquake mechanisms, magnitude, and the like, neither the damage the 1868 temblor caused nor the drama of the 1872 event seemed to compare with accounts from the New Madrid sequence, which

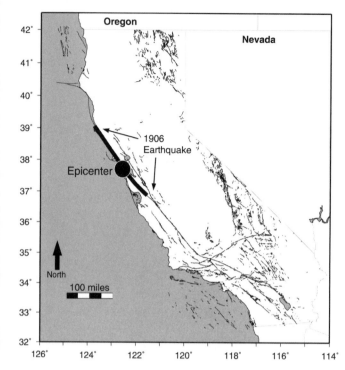

The northern San Andreas fault with the extent of the 1906 rupture indicated. The precise location of the epicenter is somewhat uncertain, but seismologists think it was near the marked location.

described large tracts of land sinking and the Mississippi River temporarily reversing its course.

Authors who write nonfiction books about subjects such as history and science might well be moved to say a silent prayer: please don't let me be proved wrong before, or shortly after, my book is published. But rarely are authors proved as spectacularly wrong as was Mr. McClellan, when only a few decades after he wrote those words the great 1906 earthquake struck San Francisco—gashing a 280-mile (500-kilometer) tear along the San Andreas fault that forever sealed California's reputation within the United States as Earthquake Country. Before discussing the temblor itself, we'll focus on a tour of the fault itself.

The San Andreas Fault

The San Andreas fault had been identified, sort of, before 1906. In 1895, geologist A. C. Lawson wrote about a "remarkably straight fault" that had "conditioned the San Andreas and Crystal Springs Valley" on the San Francisco Peninsula. However, Lawson identified only a small segment of the fault and apparently failed to recognize its significance at the time the initial work was presented. Other bits of the fault had been mapped as well, including a segment near Gorman in southern California. But nobody had connected the dots—or rather, the dashes—prior to 1906.

Following the 1906 earthquake, geologist G. K. Gilbert, accurately described the fault and the amount of slip that had occurred during the temblor, but he did not use the name San Andreas in his 1907 publication. By the time Lawson

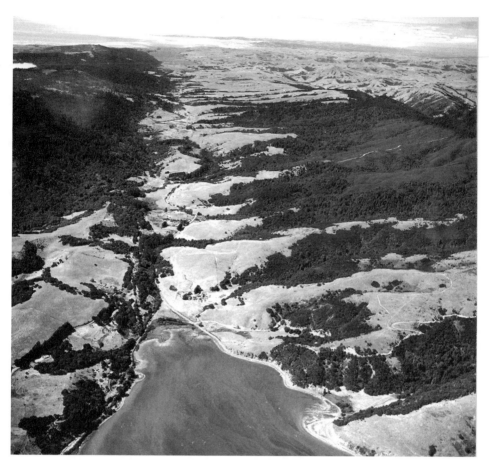

The San Andreas fault slices through Tomales Bay, viewed here toward the southeast. —ROBERT WALLACE PHOTO

published the final report of the State Earthquake Investigation Commission—the so-called Lawson Report—in 1908, the name had been adopted to describe the entirety of the fault responsible for the 1906 earthquake. (As a gossipy aside, the "A" in A. C. Lawson stood for Andrew, leading some to speculate about the extent to which he viewed the fault as, so to speak, his baby.)

In any case, the 1906 earthquake ruptured almost the full extent of the northern San Andreas fault, from San Juan Bautista in the south to just north of Shelter Cove in southern Humboldt County.

The dramatic, large-scale surface expression of the fault north of San Francisco Bay is, like so much of the fault, best appreciated from the air. We will start this part of our tour toward the fault's northern end, near Point Arena. A few miles south of where it heads offshore near Point Arena, the fault runs along the gentle valley of the Garcia River, through a wooded, sparsely populated part of the state.

Farther south, the fault makes a brief excursion offshore before reconnecting with land at Bodega Bay, where it creates a gentle scarp through the small coastal community. Here, a minor kink in fault geometry creates pressure across the fault, resulting in a subtle, linear, vertical offset. Like the Valley of the Garcia River, however, this feature is too gentle to create great visual drama at ground level. Moving southward to Tomales Bay, the fault defines a narrow, linear depression. In 1906, a maximum offset of 19 feet (6 meters) was recorded at the head of Tomales Bay, although some of this motion may have been associated with the shifting of shallow sediments.

We know today that all the territory west of the fault, including the Point Reyes Peninsula, has been carried northward hundreds of miles from southern California by continued motion along the fault over millions of years. Even before geologists were sure how much cumulative motion had occurred on the

San Andreas, they had noted the dramatic contrast between the granitic rocks of the Point Reyes Peninsula and the so-called Franciscan complex just east of Tomales Bay. The Franciscan, found along the eastern side of the San

Carol Prentice: Going to Great Lengths to Find Fault

Geologist Carol Prentice has traveled to the far ends of the earth to find faults, and her endeavors include groundbreaking (so to speak) work to identify the first known active on-land fault in Puerto Rico. She has also traveled to the far ends of North America. Her investigations of the northernmost end of the San Andreas fault have helped clarify the extent of the fault as it reaches the Mendocino Triple Junction offshore. Along much of its length, the San Andreas fault is relatively easy to find; very typically, finding faults is much more difficult at their ends, where they start to die out or trail off underwater. Yet understanding the full geometry of a fault is critical for predicting the maximum size earthquake it can generate. The work Prentice and her colleagues are doing to understand the detailed geometry of the northern terminus of the San Andreas is moreover critical to understanding the complex and evolving geometry of the Mendocino Triple Junction offshore.

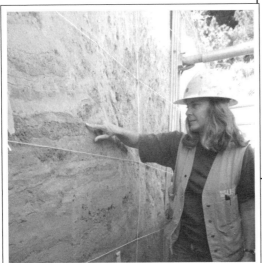

Geologist Carol Prentice points out a fault in one of the many fault trenches that she has dug and investigated during her career.

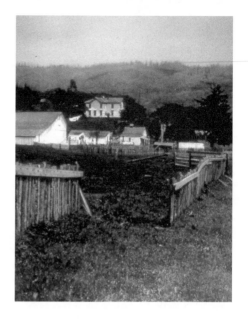

Surface rupture associated
with the 1906 San Francisco
earthquake —NOAA/NGDC PHOTO

Andreas fault for much of its northern extent, represents the detritus of California's earlier geologic history of subduction.

The subtlety of fault features belies that the stretch of fault north of San Francisco was indeed torn asunder by the 1906 earthquake. The earthquake left a dramatic, conspicuous tear that continued for hundreds of miles across the landscape. In many places, the fault offset roads and other features, leaving no doubt about the substantial lateral translation of real estate. In the immediate aftermath of the temblor, finding faults in northern California was like shooting fish in a barrel. So compelling were the observations that they led H. F. Reid to formulate the so-called elastic rebound theory of earthquake rupture (see chapter 2). First published in 1910, the theory remains one of the most fundamental tenets of earthquake science.

The 1857 Fort Tejon earthquake left a similar surface rupture, one whose lateral offset was also noted and in some cases measured by scientifically inclined observers. Elastic rebound theory might, therefore, have been developed fifty years sooner, but the fields of seismology and earthquake geology were nearly nonexistent in the 1850s, so the setting was not yet ripe for major advancements in understanding. The field of modern seismology was to a large extent born during the half century that elapsed between the two great earthquakes. In the late nineteenth century, the founding fathers of seismology, working in the United States, Japan, and Europe, first began to design and build instruments to record the waves from earthquakes. Kicking off a tradition that continues to this day, new data very quickly begot new ideas and new theories.

I digress—but for a reason. Returning to our fault tour, the salient point is that the 1906 surface rupture, a striking feature and watershed scientific data

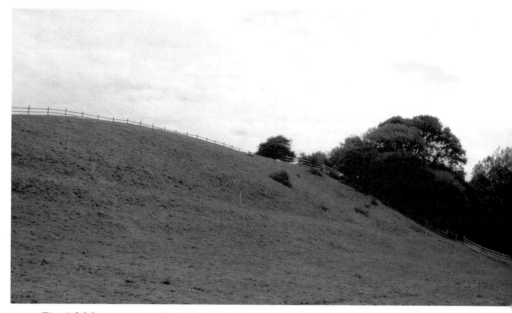

The 1906 rupture—still visible at this site—snakes along a hillside near the Earthquake Trail at the Bear Valley Visitor Center of Point Reyes National Seashore near Olema. The 1906 rupture is visible as a small, linear groove running horizontally about midway up the hillside. This site was part of the private Skinner Ranch at the time of the 1906 earthquake. (38 02.51N 122 47.81W)

set in its day, has been all but erased by the ravages of time. We can still find the fault easily enough, but, for the most part, only by looking for relatively gentle, large-scale features. Time and the elements have long since softened, if not erased any hint of recent breakage.

However, some evidence remains of the surface break in many locations. While subtle to the untrained eye, the features are striking to a geologist. One such location is on the site of the former Skinner Ranch, now part of the Point Reyes National Seashore, on the Point Reyes peninsula north of San Francisco. An earthquake trail leads visitors along a stretch of the 1906 rupture. We can reach this part of the fault by taking Francis Drake Road west from U.S. 101 or by taking California 1 from the north side of the Golden Gate Bridge. Follow the signs to the Bear Valley Visitor Center. The earthquake trail begins just south of the main parking lot. Wooden posts mark the 1906 break along the trail, which also features reconstructions of a fence offset by the rupture and of a barn that the quake knocked askew—but not over—when the rupture ran directly underneath it.

Heading southward from the Bear Valley Visitor Center, we arrive at the small town of Olema. Along the stretch of Bear Valley near Olema, the San Andreas fault is typically a rift zone a few hundred yards wide. Scientists have identified a number of fault strands and geologically recent ruptures within this zone. The San Andreas fault zone is similarly broad, comprising multiple distinct traces at

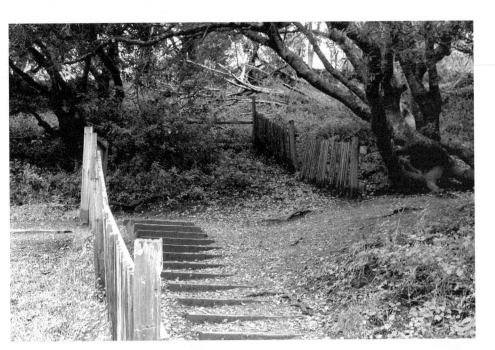

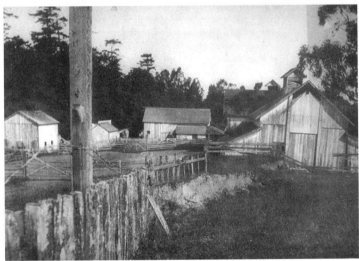

Top: A reconstructed wood fence along the Earthquake Trail reflects the amount of slip that occurred at this location in 1906, and it depicts the scene as it might have looked in the immediate aftermath of the earthquake. Note the twisted limbs of the tree in the background—this tree has clearly had a hard life growing within the San Andreas fault zone. (38 02.46N 122 47.49W)

Bottom: This historic photo was taken in 1906, where the Earthquake Trail passes today. It shows the 1906 rupture, the main trace of which ran directly beneath the barn at Skinner Ranch. —KARL V. STEINBRUGGE COLLECTION, EARTHQUAKE ENGINEERING RESEARCH CENTER

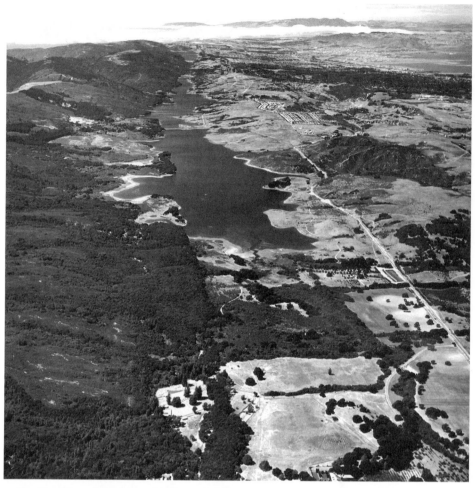

South of San Francisco, the Crystal Springs reservoir follows the San Andreas fault. The 1906 rupture ran along the left (west) side of the reservoir in the foreground. —ROBERT WALLACE PHOTO

many other locations, although here and elsewhere the 1906 rupture itself was quite narrow. One fault strand—not the main 1906 break—runs just east of California 1 near Olema, along the base of a small hill. This fault skirts the western edge of the Olema cemetery, the fenced perimeter of which we can reach by a short dirt road leading away from the highway approximately half a mile south of the intersection with Francis Drake Road. Here, the main 1906 break is west of the highway. As we continue along the valley, the 1906 rupture and the highway remain close and intertwined.

At the head of Bolinas Bay, the fault plays its last game of hide-and-seek with the Pacific Ocean, disappearing underwater one last time. Driving in towards Bolinas Bay along California 1, we are afforded a lovely view of the end of the bay and the rift valley the San Andreas fault formed—although this stretch of highway demands a driver's full attention, its curves as abundant as they are tight.

The fault remains underwater and therefore difficult to find, until it reappears on land south of San Francisco at Daly City. The fault then continues through the San Francisco peninsula—although not, we should note, through the city of San Francisco itself. This happenstance very likely spared the city from even greater damage in 1906. Instead, the fault generally traverses the valley that lies adjacent to the hilly spine of the peninsula, a valley now pressed into service to form the Crystal Springs and San Andreas reservoirs.

Although subtle, the features along the peninsula segment are dramatic enough to catch the eye even at ground level. It should come as no surprise that it is easy to find faults on the San Francisco peninsula. This is, after all, where the San Andreas fault was first identified.

Leaving San Francisco by way of I-280, we follow the valleys where Andrew Lawson first identified the "remarkably straight" fault. In Lawson's day, the valley was home to a modest lake. The original lake was dammed to create Upper and Lower Crystal Springs reservoirs, which we skirt along I-280. California 92, which we'll take west away from I-280 toward Half Moon Bay, passes between Upper and Lower Crystal Springs reservoirs. Legal stopping points are few and far between on 92, and quickly moving cars and trucks are legion. The earthquake tourist should also take note: westbound travelers on California 92 cannot turn around until climbing up the valley to a vista point on the left, several miles beyond the reservoirs.

The inner ridge of the peninsula is, fortunately, relatively sparsely populated. Still, the fault runs disturbingly close to some of the most heavily populated, not to mention some of the most expensive, real estate in the state, including not only the city of San Francisco but also San Mateo, Palo Alto, Sunnyvale, and San Jose. The pastoral Stanford University campus, nestled against the foothills a mile or two west of neighboring Palo Alto, is closer still.

One of the most convenient routes to finding faults on the peninsula is via Page Mill Road out of Palo Alto. Page Mill Road meanders just over 7 miles up through the hills, another narrow, winding road that demands one's full attention behind the wheel. We can identify the main trace of the fault by an abrupt dip in the road approximately 0.2 mile before we arrive at the Monte Bello and Los Trancos Open Space Preserves, to the left and right of Page Mill Road, respectively. The fault crossing is easier to recognize on the way down from Los Trancos than on the way up. Before we have our bearings, it is hard to tell the San Andreas fault from any other dip in the road.

Free trail guides available at the entrance to both preserves help the earthquake tourist find and understand fault features such as sag ponds and ridges

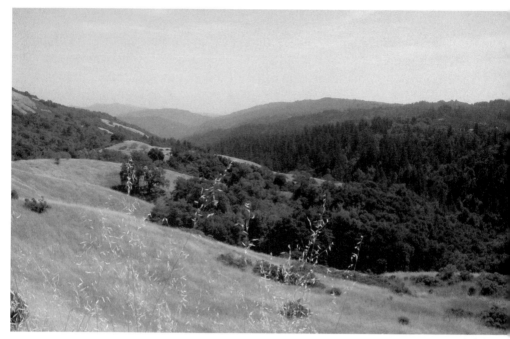

From the Monte Bello Open Space Preserve above Palo Alto, the San Andreas fault heads southward along Steven's Creek. The middle peak in the distance is Loma Prieta. (37 19.46N 122 10.67W)

formed by cross-fault compression. If the drive up Page Mill Road seems arduous, rest assured that there is gold at the end of the rainbow: arguably one of the best locations in the state to find fault.

Following the trail away from the Monte Bello parking lot, we arrive very quickly at a vantage point overlooking Stevens Creek, a fault valley whose linear character has been shaped by the San Andreas. If we let our gaze follow the valley to the mountain peaks off in the distance, on a clear day we can see Loma Prieta, which lent its lilting name to the 1989 temblor. The stretch of fault leading up to Loma Prieta is best appreciated at a distance: the terrain leading to the mountain is rugged and carpeted with poison oak.

If the Monte Bello Preserve affords a terrific view of large-scale fault features, we only need cross the street to find marvelous examples of small-scale fault features. In Los Trancos Preserve, a 1.5-mile earthquake trail provides a vantage point from which we can see Loma Prieta back toward the south. Moving along the trail, we come to a view of North Crystal Spring Reservoir and San Andreas Lake.

The best, however, is yet to come. Farther along, the trail meanders around the break of the 1906 earthquake, which is marked by yellow-banded wooden posts. (Posts with white bands mark secondary faulting.) Among the myriad earthquake sites farther along the trail is a fence that crosses the fault, reconstructed from vintage material to provide a recreation of how the scene would

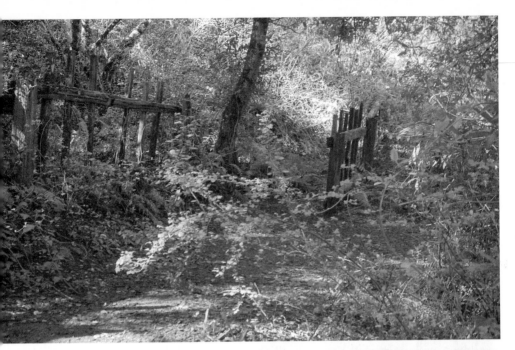

Top: Along the earthquake trail at Los
Trancos Open Space Preserve above Palo
Alto, a reconstructed fence indicates the
amount of slip that occurred at this section
of the fault in 1906.
(37 19.62N 122 10.61W)

Bottom: Researchers think the 1906 San
Francisco earthquake knocked over, but did
not kill, this tree in Los Trancos Open Space
Preserve. With its root system still intact, a
former branch that (presumably) grew after
the earthquake became a trunk and the
original main trunk eventually bent and
grew upward again as a second trunk.
(37 19.69N 122 10.71W)

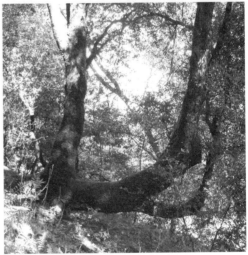

have looked immediately after the 1906 earthquake. At another point along the
trail, we arrive at soggy ground underfoot and a small sag pond; along this segment
the fault blocks the flow of groundwater, forcing it to burble to the surface.

One of the trail's stops presents the earthquake tourist with a pair of California
oak trees unlike any other. The growth pattern of these large, nearly horizontal
trunks is by no means typical for these trees. Geologists believe that the 1906
earthquake toppled these oaks but left enough of their root systems intact for
them to survive. New branches grew directly upward, and the original main trunk
eventually bent skyward as well.

The drama of these features notwithstanding, time has again softened features that were jagged and raw immediately after the great temblor struck. During a quiet period of the earthquake cycle, this trail evokes a sense of pastoral tranquility, with gentle winds and inviting forestland. To the geologically trained eye, ample evidence suggests the presence of a well-developed fault zone. Even the earth scientist, however, can find it difficult to reconcile the serenity of the area with the sheer power of the forces that have shaped it. As we stand atop one of the most impressive and hazardous major plate boundaries in the world, the warm and amiable setting beckons us to spend a few hours enjoying the California sun. Not a bad microcosm, perhaps, of the state and fault system as a whole.

Following the fault south-southwest as the crow flies away from the San Francisco Bay region, we soon reach the rugged landscape of the southern Santa Cruz Mountains. In this craggy terrain, finding faults is not easy even immediately after a great earthquake. Following the 1906 earthquake, evidence of motion along the Santa Cruz Mountains segment of the fault was both difficult to trace and, apparently, minimal. Stanford University geologist J. C. Branner sent beginning graduate student G. A. Waring to map the fault in this poison-oak-infested region. (And to think professors get accused of letting their grad students do the dirty work!) Many decades later, geologists from the U.S. Geological Survey in Menlo Park examined Waring's observations in detail and concluded that not only were most of the hapless student's observations nowhere near the fault, but he had also managed to miss a stretch of rupture a full 12 miles (20 kilometers) long. As far as modern geologists have been able to discern, the slip along this section of the fault was considerably smaller than elsewhere—but rupture indeed occured along this section of the fault.

In the late 1980s, a working group composed of eminent geologists and seismologists took on the daunting task of assessing the probability of earthquakes along the San Andreas fault's many segments. Although they reached consensus in most cases, they essentially split their vote on the Santa Cruz Mountains segment. One school of thought held that an earthquake along this segment was unlikely because the 1906 earthquake had ruptured it so recently. Another equally compelling school of thought argued that the fault had not slipped nearly as much along the Loma Prieta segment in 1906 as it had elsewhere on the fault; hence, the probability of an earthquake was quite high. Scientists belonging to the latter school were probably inclined to feel vindicated when the M6.9 Loma Prieta earthquake struck in 1989, apparently on this segment of the fault.

However, the Loma Prieta earthquake, better known in some quarters as the World Series earthquake, proved vexing beyond all expectation. Although damage was largely concentrated along soft sediment sites around San Francisco Bay, the rupture itself was nearly 50 miles (80 kilometers) away from San Francisco.

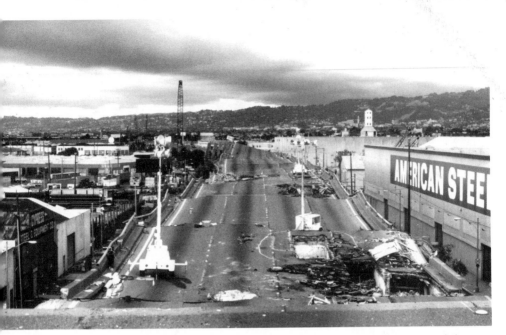

This view from the uncollapsed upper deck of the Nimitz Freeway looks toward the section of the double-deck freeway that pancaked during shaking from the 1989 Loma Prieta earthquake.

In California, an earthquake as large as Loma Prieta can generally be counted on to rupture a fault clear up to the surface, leaving a feature that geologists investigate in detail to glean important details about the rupture process. But when scientists rushed to the mountainous region to map the expected surface rupture, they found none. Instead geologists found only what they term secondary features—cracks, slumping, and other disruptions not caused by primary fault rupture. Some of these features closely mimicked those documented in the area in 1906.

Did the Loma Prieta quake really occur on the San Andreas fault at all? Immediately after the earthquake, the answer seemed obvious. The location and orientation, or strike, of the rupture appeared to place the event squarely on the mapped trace of the fault. However, detailed seismological analyses revealed not the lateral (strike-slip) motion expected for San Andreas earthquakes but rather a significant component of vertical slip. The new data also shifted the epicenter several miles west of the surface trace of the San Andreas. The Loma Prieta rupture itself was moreover not vertical, but rather dipped towards the west. Eventually, many geologists came to the conclusion that the rupture occurred not on the San Andreas fault but rather on a nearby, associated fault.

Given the rugged terrain, the substantial rates of rainfall and erosion, and the complexity of the faults in the region, it's not surprising that it is so difficult

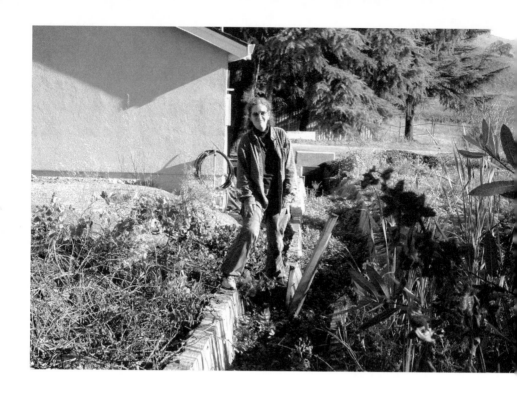

to find faults in the Santa Cruz Mountains. But rest assured, they are there. The fact was not only proved twice within a single century; it is also manifest in the landscape around Santa Cruz, where compression caused by a bend in the San Andreas fault has created a dramatic set of uplifted marine terraces.

South from the Santa Cruz Mountains region, the San Andreas emerges into more gentle terrain. The fault trace forms a small scarp along the northeastern edge of San Juan Bautista, a small farming community with a seismological claim to fame: it was here, or at least very close to here, that the 1906 rupture terminated.

San Juan Bautista remains at a crossroads today as well. South of the town, the San Andreas fault is not locked but instead moves gradually, or creeps. Creeping faults do not store energy in the manner described by elastic rebound theory. Instead they move gradually and steadily, producing an ongoing smattering of small earthquakes, a few moderate ones (M4 to M5), but no large events. For reasons not entirely understood, creeping faults are rare. The approximately 125-mile (200-kilometer) segment of the San Andreas fault southeast of San Juan Bautista is one of the most striking examples of a creeping fault anywhere on earth.

Creeping faults might be more benign than their locked brethren, but they do sometimes pose special challenges. Just south of San Juan Bautista, the owners of the DeRose winery face these challenges constantly. Part of the winery (formerly the Almaden-Cienega winery) was built directly atop the creeping fault—and the building's walls are paying the price for their inopportune location. The winery,

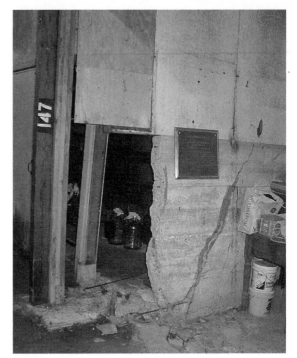

Left: The author stands atop culvert immediately south of the DeRose winery. The culvert has been offset by creep along the San Andreas fault. Famous for decades in geology circles as the Almaden-Cienega winery, the winery was sold to the DeRose family in 1988.

Right: DeRose winery building reveals damage to wall and floor caused by creep on the San Andreas fault.

which is nestled within a lovely valley and makes an equally lovely cabernet, is a short drive from central Hollister, about 6.5 miles south on Cienega Road from the corner of Cienega and Union Roads.

This chapter's tour of the San Andreas fault will come to a close at this point, leaving discussion of the central segment of the fault for the following chapter. It is perhaps sobering to look back over the segment of the fault we have traversed so far in this chapter: a stretch nearly 300 miles long, the full extent of which ruptured in the great 1906 earthquake. Painstaking geologic investigations have shown that over the long haul, this northern segment moves about an inch per year. This value does not represent the total amount of plate motion, but it certainly accounts for the lion's share. And now that our tour of the fault itself is finished, it is time to discuss the earthquake that made the fault famous.

The Big One: 1906

The 1906 earthquake not only taught seismologists much of what we know about great strike-slip earthquakes, but also serves as an archetype for the "Big One"— the large earthquake that eventually will occur again on the San Andreas fault.

The first rumblings on April 18, 1906, started at 5:12 A.M., local time, when a moderate earthquake was felt widely throughout the San Francisco Bay Area. Although people had commonly felt small-to-moderate earthquakes in the region through the last half of the nineteenth century, this modest temblor would prove to be different—it was a foreshock. Foreshocks are somewhat vexing creatures

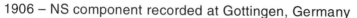
1906 – NS component recorded at Gottingen, Germany

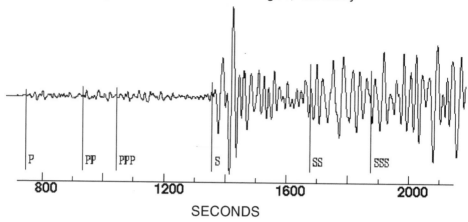

| P | PP | PPP | | S | | SS | | SSS |

800   1200   1600   2000

SECONDS

Seismogram of the 1906 San Francisco earthquake recorded in Germany

to seismologists. As far as we can tell, they are nothing more than garden-variety earthquakes. They appear to stand apart from the vast majority (about 95 percent) of their brethren only by virtue of the fact that they are followed by events larger than themselves. (And, yes, this after-the-fact definition is as unsatisfying to the scientist as it probably seems to the layperson. Unfortunately, it remains the best we can do.) After any small or moderate earthquake in California, seismologists can only resort to a statement based on the statistics of past earthquakes: there is approximately a one-in-twenty chance that any earthquake will be followed by something larger within three days.

For a few short seconds, the rumblings on the morning of April 18 would have felt no different from any of the numerous moderate earthquakes that had struck the greater San Francisco Bay Area in previous decades. But just twenty to twenty-five seconds later, all hell broke loose. The earth unleashed a singular fury, described by William Ford Nichols, the Episcopal bishop of California at the time, as "JOLT-jolt-jolt, sway-sway-sway, rattle-rattle-rattle over big, age-like tens of seconds with a deep diapason of rumbling, and then a great ugly, last BANG."

Through detailed analysis of shaking, seismologists have concluded that the earthquake initiated close to San Francisco and ruptured in both directions along the fault, southeast to San Juan Bautista and northwest to Point Arena. A small handful of early seismometers at far-flung locations around the globe recorded the temblor. These "teleseismic" instruments were designed to record the low-amplitude waves from large earthquakes at great distances—and they did indeed record waves from the 1906 earthquake.

When the northern San Andreas fault ruptures again the waves will be recorded by teleseismic instruments but also by a plethora of so-called strong-motion

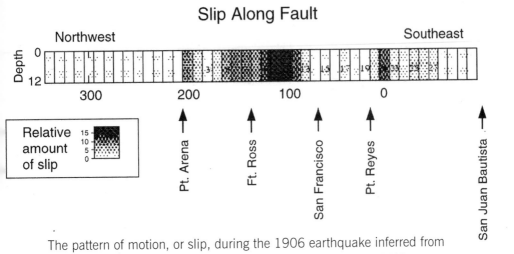

Slip Along Fault

The pattern of motion, or slip, during the 1906 earthquake inferred from analysis of available seismogram. —FROM THE WORK OF DAVID WALD

instruments within California. Several agencies operate these instruments, most notably the U.S. Geological Survey and the California Geological Survey. These instruments will record the high-amplitude shaking—every jolt, sway, rattle, and BANG—and allow seismologists to map out the distribution of shaking throughout the state. Such maps are now routinely generated following large earthquakes, such as the 1992 M7.3 Landers, California, event.

The only seismogram data available for the 1906 earthquake are the few teleseismic recordings mentioned from distant instruments. Seismologists are able to use such data to investigate the details of an earthquake, but only crudely compared to what is possible with modern data. When data from seismometers are scarce, seismologists can also turn to the distribution of damage and perceived shaking intensity documented by anecdotal accounts. Properly analyzed using calibrations established by modern earthquakes, such accounts can provide important details about an earthquake source. This approach did indeed prove useful for investigations of the 1906 earthquake.

Researchers use anecdotal accounts to assign "intensities" that reflect shaking severity. These intensity values are usually denoted by Roman numerals: from I to II for barely perceptible tremors and up to XII for near-total destruction, including collapse of modern, well-designed structures.

To determine intensity values, researchers must generally look beyond descriptions such as the portion of Bishop Nichols' account. As qualitatively descriptive as his account is, it does not provide a good indication of the severity of the jolts, sways, and rattles—let alone the rumbles and the "BANG." Scientists generally determine intensity values from more objective descriptions of effects, such as whether objects were knocked off of shelves and the extent of structural damage.

Later in his account, Bishop Nichols did include precisely the kind of information that seismologists look for: "The house had stood solidly . . . though . . . one chimney had tossed out so that the top went through our roof, and the center of . . . the roof next door; the other 2 chimney tops were moved from the base, and several courses of bricks were thrown out of the front gable." From this, we know that the shaking was strong enough to damage weaker architectural elements, such as chimneys and gables, but not strong enough to substantively damage or destroy the house.

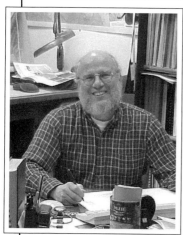

Jerry Treiman

tectonic processes and the landscape. Scientists such as Treiman use this geomorphic evidence, along with traditional geologic mapping and paleoseismic investigations, to gauge the slip-rate and recency of activity of faults in this geologically active state. As a result of these sorts of classical geological investigations, the database of known active faults in California is far more extensive than that for other regions. This knowledge translates into the ability to assess hazard at a far greater degree of detail and sophistication than is possible elsewhere.

Mapping Active Faults

The California Geological Survey, formerly the California Division of Mines and Geology, has a mandate to map active faults in the state and to assess the hazard they pose. Jerry Treiman, a geologist for twenty-five years at the California Geological Survey, has mapped not only faults but also main-shock ruptures such as the long and complex scars left by the 1992 Landers and 1999 Hector Mine earthquakes. Treiman's fascination with geology and its role in shaping landscapes formed during early hiking and camping experiences. During his student days at UCLA and his professional career at the state survey, Treiman has developed an understanding of the relationship between the

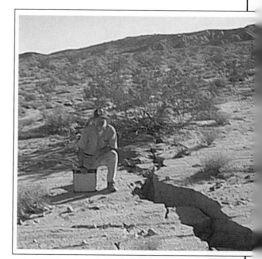

Jerry Treiman alongside the rupture of the 1999 Hector Mine earthquake, California

Given this type of information, one final piece of information remains before a seismologist can assign intensities with confidence: the type and quality of the construction. The intensity scale that most American seismologists use, the modified Mercalli intensity (MMI) scale, distinguishes between four types of construction ranging from poorly built, unreinforced masonry to wood- or steel-frame construction designed to withstand earthquake shaking. Returning to the bishop's house, we know the building was masonry (brick) and not specifically designed for earthquakes. But how well was it built? Bishop Nichols was most obliging on this score as well, noting that the architect had later examined the house, and "it had stood remarkably well, there being no structural damage, owing to its good foundation and strong and honest construction."

Few earthquake accounts are as complete as Bishop Nichols', but seismologists can still glean detailed intensity data from accounts and, for relatively recent earthquakes, photographs. The 1906 earthquake poses a special challenge because the subsequent fire destroyed so much of what the earthquake left standing, but a fair number of photographs were taken before the fire consumed the city.

Scientists made detailed intensity maps immediately after the temblor, and subsequent reexamination of original accounts has generally corroborated the

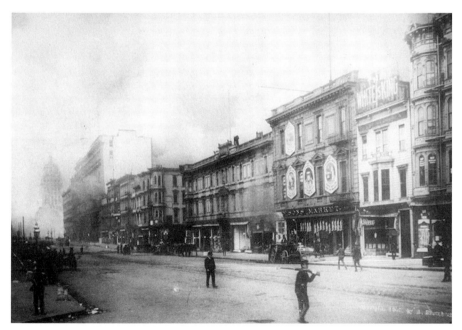

Although most photographs of the 1906 earthquake reflect damage from the fire as well as the earthquake, a relatively small number were taken before the fire took its toll on the city. Some, such as this one, indicate surprisingly low levels of damage to some buildings. —KARL V. STEINBRUGGE COLLECTION, EARTHQUAKE ENGINEERING RESEARCH CENTER

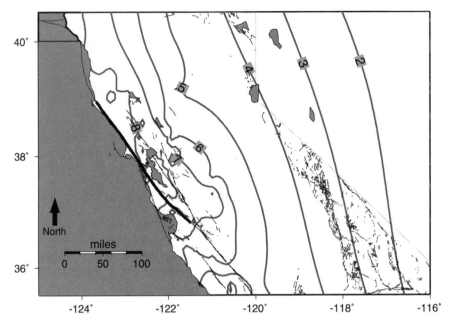

Distribution of shaking intensity during the 1906 earthquake. Contoured severity of shaking is indicated with the modified Mercalli intensity scale: high intensity values (8+) correspond to several damage while the lowest values (2 to 3) correspond to shaking that is barely perceptible to humans.
—DATA FROM TOUSSON TOPPOZADA AND DAVID BRANUM

veracity of these maps. What they show is surprising: the city of San Francisco was not reduced to rubble by the earthquake. In fact, many parts of the city suffered surprisingly light damage, sparing even the type of weak architectural elements that were damaged in the bishop's house.

Nearly one hundred years after 1906, seismologist Jack Boatwright used the accounts to develop a model for the rupture: where it started and how it progressed. He showed that the relatively light damage could be explained as, essentially, happenstance—a consequence of the detailed evolution of rupture. Like snowflakes, no two earthquakes are exactly the same, even those that rupture the same stretch of fault. Instead they leave behind uneven patterns of slip unique to every event.

In addition to the rupture model derived to fit the intensity pattern, Boatwright also constructed models with the same overall parameters (magnitude, fault location, and so forth) but with different rupture details. Some of these models produced significantly stronger shaking in the city of San Francisco, which highlights a sobering point: given the mercurial nature of earthquake wave propagation, the next Big One might cause significantly less *or more* severe shaking than the last Big One.

Along the northern San Andreas fault, the last Big One certainly seemed big enough—big enough to move 280 miles of the plate boundary and to forever seal our view of California as Earthquake Country.

Other Faults, Other Times

In any discussion of earthquake hazard in the greater Bay Area, two earthquakes inevitably dominate: 1906 and 1989. In contrast, beginning in 1971 the greater Los Angeles region was rocked by a number of Pretty Big Ones that illuminated the complexity of the region's faults and the distributed hazard associated with them. But if our awareness of Bay Area earthquake history were limited to the twentieth century, we would conclude that the San Andreas fault—and perhaps secondary faults immediately adjacent to it—are virtually the only show in town.

We would be wrong.

To understand the hazard posed by secondary faults in the northern part of the California plate-boundary system, it is helpful to first discuss some recent theoretical developments in seismology. Current models for regional earthquake activity (anywhere) involve a concept known as the earthquake cycle. According to this model, the overall rate of earthquakes on any given fault is controlled by the rate at which plate tectonics and other forces are applying stress to the system. Think of it as an energy balance: energy goes into the system as forces push blocks of crust in ways they cannot easily move; energy is released from the system when blocks lurch past one another in earthquakes. In its most simple incarnation, such a theory predicts why a fault such as the San Andreas produces earthquakes every two hundred years, give or take, while a given fault in New York or Oklahoma might produce big earthquakes every 50,000 years (give or take a few tens of thousands of years).

More recently, however, scientists have developed a more complex model of an earthquake cycle, one with two key features. First, large earthquakes are now known to affect the occurrence of other earthquakes by virtue of their ability to redistribute stress. Second, the modern models for the earthquake cycle describe not only the occurrence of large earthquakes but also the rates of small and moderate events before and after the Big Ones. This second aspect of the model has particularly important implications for the psychology of earthquakes—that is, the way that people perceive earthquakes and earthquake hazards. And the San Francisco Area provides a prime case in point.

Before discussing the Bay Area's faults, though, let me say a bit more about the theories in general. Returning to the idea of an earthquake budget, we find that big earthquakes can increase the stress on immediately adjacent faults. Although complex in detail, this phenomenon is conceptually straightforward. In general, however, recall that big earthquakes take stored energy *out* of the system. Following a large earthquake, therefore, we can think of the local stored energy

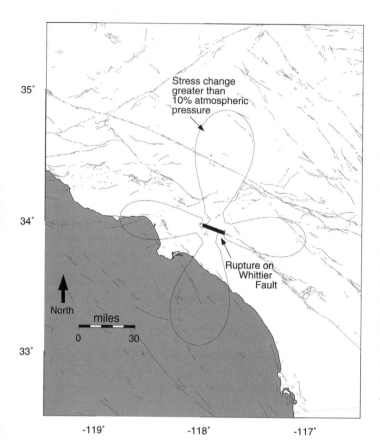

Every earthquake affects the stress in the crust surrounding the part of the fault that moved. The four-lobed contour here shows the predicted stress change from a theoretical earthquake on the northern end of the Whittier fault, east of the city of Los Angeles. Within this contour, stress increases by 0.1 bar, an amount equivalent to one-tenth of atmospheric pressure. Seismologists generally consider stress changes of this magnitude and higher sufficient to trigger aftershocks. —WORK BY JEANNE HARDEBECK

Stress change greater than 10% atmospheric pressure

Rupture on Whittier Fault

North

miles

0   30

clock being reset to zero. As time marches forward, stresses begin to accumulate again, but at first these stresses are small and unevenly distributed throughout the crust. In such a state, the crust generates relatively few small and moderate earthquakes. Earth scientists use the phrase, "stress shadow" to describe the effect a large earthquake has on regional seismicity over the years or decades following the large event.

Eventually, however, stress shadows begin to erode. Stress builds up not only on large faults but also in surrounding regions. Seismologists talk in terms of the "correlation" of a stress field—another idea that is conceptually quite straight-forward. Imagine a machine that blows soap bubbles over a small pond (no, really!). Just after the machine is turned on, individual soap bubbles will land on the water and linger only briefly before popping. The effect on the pond will be small, lim-ited to isolated soap splotches. But if the machine stays on for a long time, and generates bubbles fast enough, eventually the bubbles will land atop one another and begin to coalesce. The splotches will grow bigger, eventually reaching out to touch neighboring splotches until the pond is one big pool of soap scum. This is what scientists mean by spatial *correlation*: the degree to which something is clumped, as opposed to random.

Stress in the crust works the same way—sort of. Large-scale forces, not bubble-blowing forces, generate seismic stress. But because of the complexity of the crust, seismologists think stress accumulates unevenly, with pockets of stress developing in a manner similar to the aggregation of bubbles. Early in the cycle, high-stress pockets might exist where previous earthquakes happened to leave isolated patches of leftover stress. According to current models, the crust moves progressively from a relaxed state immediately after a large earthquake to a state in which the stress field increases both in amplitude and degree of correlation—that is, the stress becomes more intense and the clumps of high stress grow larger in area. Eventually the crust is ready to support another large earthquake, but before that happens it begins to generate more frequent small and moderate earthquakes. Hence, the more complex image of an earthquake cycle: one in which smaller events start to occur more frequently, presaging (by perhaps decades) future large events.

Now reintroduce people into the equation. By necessity, human beings approach life through an ongoing process of triage, focusing their attentions and energies on the problems, issues, and people immediately at hand. Seismologists express perennial frustration at society's short collective memory for earthquakes. People *should* take a more long-term view of earthquake hazard, and one of the more important roles that the earth scientist plays is to swim against the inexorable tide of human nature. But inevitably, out of sight—and out of recent memory—is out of mind where earthquakes are concerned.

And in the greater San Francisco Bay Area, earthquakes have been largely out of sight throughout the twentieth century. Loma Prieta may still loom large in collective memory, but felt earthquakes were, on the whole, fairly rare beasts during this particular one-hundred-year period.

Such was not always the case. The Museum of San Francisco Web site maintains a treasure trove of information about historic earthquakes. Among its electronically archived documents are lists of felt earthquakes dating back to California's mission and ranchero days. The early records are somewhat uneven, but the tally becomes more complete at the start of the Gold Rush in 1849.

To give just a few examples, six earthquakes were felt in 1858, including the one that damaged city hall in San Francisco and caused "much damage" in San Jose. The following year a dozen earthquakes were felt. In 1865, more than twenty earthquakes were felt, including one on October 8 that caused significant damage. Just three years later, an even larger earthquake struck on October 21. (Later in this chapter, we'll investigate this temblor, known at the time as the great 1868 San Francisco earthquake.)

Seismologists cannot generally estimate the magnitudes of historic earthquakes with great precision, but researchers think the 1865 and 1868 earthquakes were of M6.5 and M7.0, respectively. The myriad small events probably ranged in size

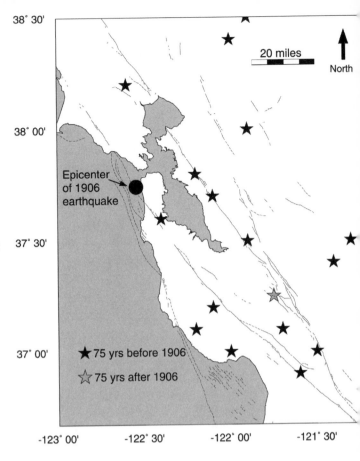

Black stars indicate the earthquakes of M6.0 or greater that struck the San Francisco Bay Area during the seventy-five years prior to the 1906 earthquake. Within the same region, only a single earthquake larger than M6.0 (gray star) hit during the seventy-five years following 1906.

from M3.0 to perhaps M5.0, and they clearly popped off at a more prodigious rate through the mid-1800s than during the late 1900s. According to what we now know (or think we know) about earthquake cycles, these fluctuations were not simply random. The San Andreas fault in northern California was nearing the end of its cycle, producing small, moderate, and even a few large earthquakes on the San Andreas and on other regional faults.

The same process appears to have also played out on a smaller scale in the years before the Loma Prieta earthquake. An increased smattering of small and moderate events, although fewer in number than those that came before 1906, preceded this earthquake. It was, however, observations of the pre-1989 seismicity that first led seismologists toward modern theories of earthquake cycles. Only later did researchers turn their attention to the more dramatic events of the previous century and recognize a similar pattern.

The latter half of the nineteenth century provides a dramatic illustration of the hazard associated with Bay Area faults other than the San Andreas. These faults may be especially active in the decades preceding great San Andreas fault earthquakes, but they are certainly capable of producing damaging earthquakes at other times as well. In the following sections we'll explore several of the other larger—and potentially most damaging—faults in and around the greater San Francisco Bay Area.

The Hayward Fault

If the northern San Andreas fault were a tree trunk, the Hayward fault would be one of its largest branches—the one that would demolish your car were it broken off in a storm. In map view, the fault even appears branchlike. And the analogy is equally apt when one considers its damage potential.

A set of faults veers eastward away from the San Andreas fault near San Juan Bautista, beginning with the Calaveras fault. The Calaveras is perhaps best known for its ability to move—at least in the shallow crust—by means of the steady process of creep. As we'll soon see, the small town of Hollister, which the Calaveras fault neatly bisects, has traditionally provided many of the textbook examples of a fault creep.

The Hayward fault splays back westward from the Calaveras near Milpitas, near where California 237 intersects I-680. From its point of origin, the fault runs northwesterly—directly through the heart of the densely populated East Bay. Fremont, Hayward, Oakland, Berkeley—these modern-day boomtowns are strewn like pearls along the fault strand until it disappears under San Pablo Bay. What happens to it at this juncture is an interesting question unto itself, and one that we will return to shortly.

But first the storied history of the Hayward fault itself. Before 1906, the Great San Francisco Earthquake had not struck San Francisco at all, but rather had occurred on the Hayward fault on the morning of October 21, 1868. The temblor ruptured about a 15-mile (25-kilometer) segment of the fault between Oakland and Fremont, and seismologists now estimate its magnitude at approximately 7.0, large enough to leave a wide wake of damage in both San Francisco and the East Bay.

Presaging observations that would be made more than once again in the twentieth century, an article in the *San Francisco Morning Call* observed that buildings west of Montgomery Street escaped relatively unscathed, while "east of Montgomery, upon that portion which has been reclaimed from the Bay and is called 'new-made ground,' the damage was considerable."

By 1868, San Francisco was a booming city. As Rolander McClellan described it in *The Golden State*, "The floodgates of commerce and population were [opened after 1849], and through them poured a torrent of human beings upon the little village of San Francisco, with its few adobe and frame houses." Two decades later the village had become a thriving urban center.

San Francisco had also experienced damaging ground shaking often enough that the potential effect on property values had not escaped the attention of the city's property owners and speculators—nor had the potential for even greater disasters than those experienced previously. In 1867, an issue of *The San Francisco Real Estate Circular* noted that "many old ladies of the male sex have often allowed their foolish fears to take the form of prophesies, that San Francisco would some time or other be totally destroyed by [an earthquake]." But even in the aftermath of the 1868 temblor—the so-called Great San Francisco Earthquake—*The San Francisco Real Estate Circular* sagely concluded, "Even, therefore, if San Francisco was visited by a calamitous earthquake, its progressive career as a city would be but temporarily interrupted, and though real estate and other values might suffer from an immediate panic, they would quickly recover again."

Sentiments such as these may sound cavalier in retrospect, but the reality is that earthquake risk mitigation has continued to be predicated on the concept of "acceptable risk." As a rule, acceptable risk has included appreciable (tolerable) property losses as long as human safety is ensured. The concept is by no means as alien as it may seem. After all, automobile makers don't design cars to come through accidents unscathed but rather to protect their human occupants.

However, as cities grow so, too, does risk. With real estate inventories in modern megacities now approaching values measured in trillions, risk previously considered acceptable may well be too costly to bear. The most damaging United States earthquake to date, the Northridge quake, left an estimated thirty billion dollars in total property damage—and it was only a Pretty Big One. It was also largely a glancing blow—its most severe shaking occurred away from the population centers. We can no longer ignore the potential risk from a true Big One and/or a more direct hit on a population center. A price tag of one hundred billion dollars (or more) in direct losses is difficult to accept—especially when estimation scenarios of loss predict accompanying human death tolls numbering well into the thousands.

In several megacities, therefore, local, state, and federal governments have taken some fairly remarkable steps in recent years to reduce potential losses of property—as well as human life. We can find many examples of mitigation in the East Bay, particularly on the Hayward fault. To illustrate this point, let's now move on to the next stop on our fault tour.

Finding Fault in the East Bay

Finding fault in the East Bay is fairly easy because, at least at shallow depths, the Hayward fault now creeps at a fairly healthy clip, approximately 0.1 to 0.5 inch (0.3 to 1 centimeter) per year. In this case, seismologists think creep does not obviate hazard because they think the fault is locked at depth. The creep does, however, leave little doubt where the fault is. Consider it something of a bad news–good news situation.

It is only fitting to begin an earthquake tour of the East Bay in Fremont, near the southern terminus of the 1868 rupture. From I-680, the Durham Road/Auto Mall Parkway exit provides a convenient route east to the fault, which is generally

Top: The Hayward fault through the East Bay Area. Circles indicate locations of some of the photographs in this chapter: two each in Fremont and Hayward, and two (from the same location) in Berkeley.

Bottom: At the Fremont Christian Life Center in Fremont, the Hayward fault cuts across the parking lot and passes beneath one of the church buildings. Here the author is standing where fault creep has gradually offset the parking lot curb. (37 30.88N 121 56.24W)

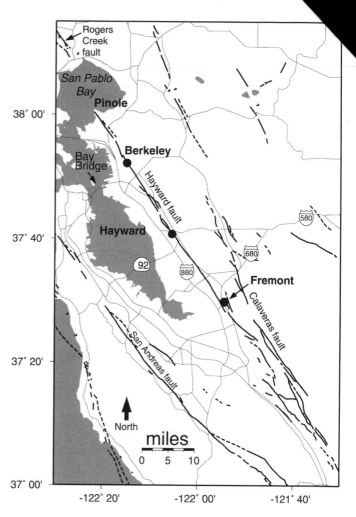

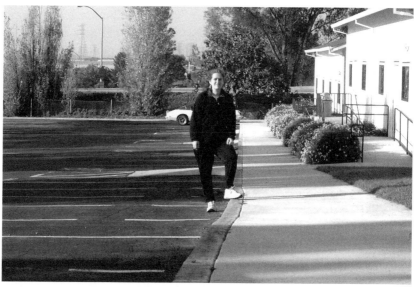

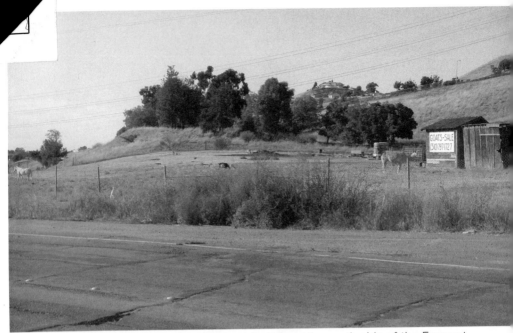

In this view north along the Hayward fault from the north side of the Fremont Christian Life Center, the fault creates a low scarp that cuts through a pen of farm animals. The fault also cuts across the road, which shows evidence of cracking and repair. (37 30.89N 121 56.24W)

defined in the East Bay by a small but abrupt vertical offset that roughly parallels I-680. Heading east from the freeway on Durham Road, we reach the fault when we arrive at the first intersection. On the northeast corner of the intersection, the fault's handiwork stands as a small hill. On the southeast corner, we find a small church, the parking lot of which proves that, well, even churches have their faults. The Hayward fault cuts diagonally across the church parking lot, leaving the telltale series of cracks in the asphalt and disruptions in curbs and sidewalks. Heading north away from the church, the fault crosses and chews up Durham Road before continuing through an open field with goats for sale. (At some point, these goats and their pasture will likely give way to development and no longer serve as a landmark for finding fault.)

Continuing up Durham Road approximately 0.4 mile to Paseo Padre Parkway, we can turn south and proceed another 0.5 mile to Grimmer Road. A quick right onto Grimmer leads quickly to an intersection that the Hayward fault diagonally bisects, disrupting asphalt once again and doing unfriendly things to houses unfortunate enough to sit immediately atop the fault trace.

Returning to Grimmer and driving west approximately 0.5 mile, we arrive at Warm Springs Road, which, heading northward, becomes Osgood Avenue after crossing the intersection with Auto Mall Parkway. Along this stretch of road, Osgood

Avenue is nearly right on top of the fault. We can see fault effects just east of the road, typically in the form of hills or ridges.

About 1.8 miles north of the Auto Mall Parkway, we arrive at the corner of Osgood and Washington Avenues. At the southeast corner of this intersection, we find a well-fenced, abandoned piece of property—the former site of the Gallegos Winery, established in 1884. The ill-fated winery (photos of which are on display in the rental store opposite the site) was heavily damaged by the 1906 earthquake, and the owners subsequently tore down the structure. The earthquake had, however, only hastened the inevitable, for the winery's thick stone walls had been built squarely atop the creeping Hayward fault. Given the creep rate that modern instruments now estimate, these walls would have been wrenched by about 3 feet (1 meter) in the century following 1906, an assault they were unlikely to withstand. The lovely and centrally located parcel of property now appears to be a sterling example of unbuildable real estate. (The parcel was actually once slated for use as a parking lot for a BART [Bay Area Rapid Transit] terminal until plans for the terminal were scrapped.)

Following the Hayward fault north of the winery, however, we find structures that were built well after 1906—but before we fully appreciated the destructive potential of both creep and earthquakes.

Leaving the Gallegos Winery site by way of Washington Boulevard, we can continue about 1.5 miles to Stevenson Road and turn right. After about a mile, we turn into a park complex at Center Drive. In the middle of Fremont Central Park, we find Lake Elizabeth. Before the human intervention, Lake Elizabeth was a swampy sag pond, in this case a small body of water that forms in the step, or jog, between two fault segments. All long faults include myriad disruptions such as kinks and small "step overs." Such disruptions manifest in characteristic

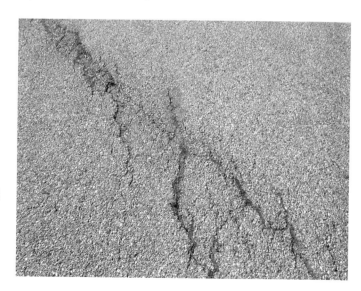

At the corner of Grimmer and Gardenia Avenues (two residential streets in Fremont), the creeping Hayward fault trace cuts diagonally across the intersection, leaving behind a telltale pattern of cracks in the pavement. (37 30.48N 121 55.87W)

that we can understand through simple geometrical considerations. Recall ..... a jog in a strike-slip fault will cause either a small region of compression or one of extension, depending on the direction of the jog and the motion on the fault.

In Fremont, city officials expanded the sag pond into a small lake that now lies within a large municipal complex and park. With gently rolling expanses of green and the picturesque lake, the complex reflects the best of civic intentions—

Roger Bilham and the Creep Meters

Roger Bilham's investigations have taken him to the far corners of the globe many times over, including destinations such as Mount Kilimanjaro, Mount Everest, and Tibet. Early in his career, one of his primary interests was building elegantly simple scientific instruments to record, among other things, the steady process of fault creep. Some of these instruments have remained in the ground for decades, monitoring slow movements on the Hayward fault and along the San Andreas fault. (Among these locations is the former site of the Gallegos Winery; the 1906 earthquake destroyed the structure, but creep continues to shift remaining parts of walls.) If faults do start to slip slowly before large earthquakes, as some scientists and anecdotal evidence suggests, this process may someday be caught by creep meters. At Parkfield, where anecdotal evidence suggests that a creep episode may have preceded the moderate 1966 Parkfield earthquake, creep meters should someday provide a definitive answer to the question.

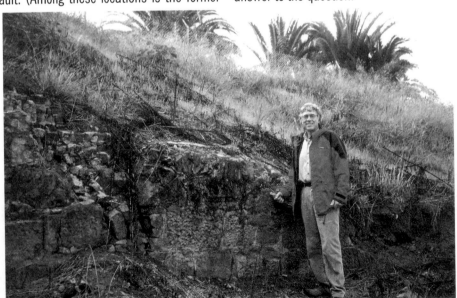

Roger Bilham stands in front of a remaining section of a wall from the former Gallegos Winery that has been rotated from its original position by continued creep on the Hayward fault.

intentions unfortunately gone awry. The city constructed a new, modern town hall in the 1990s, the centerpiece of the complex. But shortly thereafter, geologists and planners realized that the Hayward fault runs right between the structure's tall support columns. With retrofit costs deemed prohibitive, in 1998 town leaders made a decision to build a new city hall elsewhere. Today the complex is used as a park, by city police, and as home to the Fremont public library, which was judged to be far enough from the trace of the fault to remain in use. Overall, however, the complex conveys the impression of a modern-day ghost town, abandoned not when the gold ran out, but when ignorance gave way to understanding.

From Fremont Central Park, we can head farther east on Stevenson to Mission Boulevard, which heads north approximately 8 miles before reaching the city of Hayward. Driving through Union City, we parallel the fault, which lies a few short tenths of a mile west of the road. Where Mission enters the heart of downtown Hayward, we find ourselves in the middle of one of the most famous walking tours in California—famous walking fault tours, that is. This part of the tour can also be reached directly from the Hayward BART station, conveniently located just a few short blocks west of Mission.

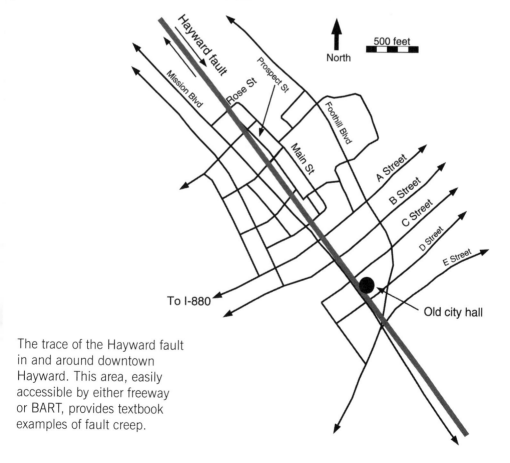

The trace of the Hayward fault in and around downtown Hayward. This area, easily accessible by either freeway or BART, provides textbook examples of fault creep.

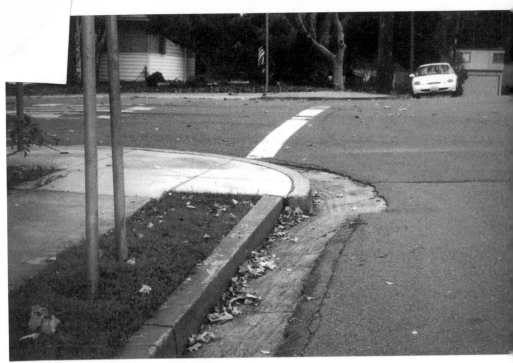

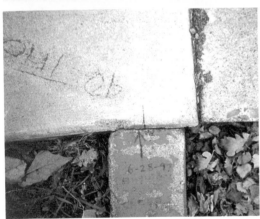

At the corner of Rose and Prospect Streets in Hayward, the Hayward fault neatly bisects sections of the curb at the northwest corner of the intersection, progressively shifting them. A line and date were drawn across the curb in 1997, *(close-up photo)* providing a datum against which we can estimate that the fault crept about 0.5 inch (1 centimeter) between 1997 and 2001, when the photograph was taken. (37 40.79N 122 05.47W)

The Hayward tour is perhaps best appreciated as a modest loop. From the corner of Mission Boulevard and B Street, walk north along Mission. The street scene itself isn't much to look at, so look instead to the east—at the short but steep hill immediately east of the road. By now it comes as no surprise that the hill is there because the fault is there.

At Rose Avenue turn right (east) and proceed up the hill to the corner of Rose and Prospect. At the northwest side of the intersection, we find one of the most photographed street curbs in the state of California, if not the world. Cleanly cut by the fault, the curb and the street are continuously offset by fault creep—until people come along to dutifully make repairs. On June 28, 1997, the curb became

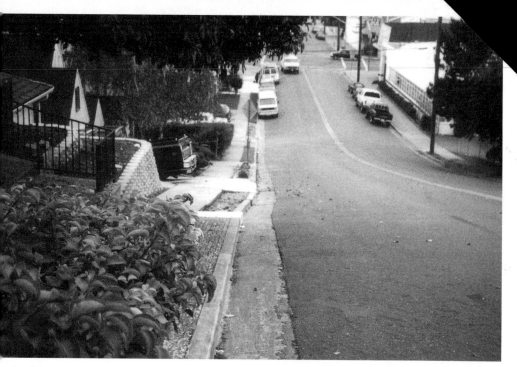

Looking west along cross streets as we walk along Prospect Avenue in Hayward, we find evidence of fault creep in the roads and sidewalks. (37 40.72N 1122 05.41W)

a makeshift creep meter when a geologically inclined soul painted a straight red line across the curb and inscribed the date.

Heading back south along Prospect, finding the fault is an interesting exercise. It does not follow the road, but rather angles back toward Mission. At most of the cross streets, therefore, the handiwork of creep is visible as the telltale warping of curbs. The offsets progress farther toward Mission as we continue along. Taking one of the cross streets, such as A Street, back to Mission and continuing south, we rejoin the fault—which then continues through the heart of the historic downtown. Finding a fault in such a quaint but heavily utilized urban setting is tricky because repairs continually erase evidence of faulting. However, fresh cracks or repairs in brick buildings sometimes indicate that the fault trace lies below.

One notable structure has remained in a steady state for many years, however: the old city hall, built directly atop the fault on the site of the Rancho San Lorenzo land grant of 1842. This structure, too, was abandoned because of damage caused by fault creep—because of untenable future repair costs. When an elegant new city hall was built in 1998, city planners took no chances, designing the structure with state-of-the-art engineering to withstand a M7.0 earthquake on the Hayward fault. Meanwhile, the old city hall remains grand, and its grounds

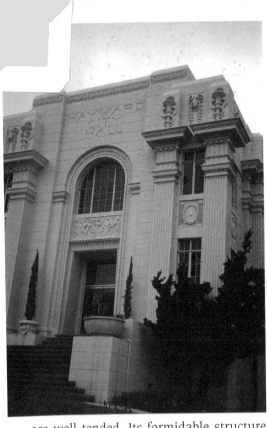

Old Hayward City Hall. The elegant building was constructed atop the creeping Hayward fault in downtown Hayward and had to be abandoned. (37 40.23N 122 04.94W)

are well tended. Its formidable structure shows little evidence of damage. Only up close can we peer through windows and recognize it for the ghostly sentinel it has become.

Following the fault farther north from Fremont, we soon arrive in Oakland, where the fault generally skirts along the base of the hills. Scientists have investigated the fault by trenching it in Montclair Park, which we can reach by taking the Thornhill Drive/Moraga Avenue exit from California 13 and heading south on Moraga Avenue. Scientists have found evidence of the 1868 rupture there along with evidence of an earlier large earthquake, perhaps between 1640 and 1776. The fault also cuts through the front entrance to the Oakland Zoo, at 37 45.12N 122 08.95W, although evidence is subtle.

In Temescal Park, near the border between Oakland and Berkeley, the fault runs through a children's playground near the southeast end of the park, leaving a telltale pattern of en echelon cracks as it cuts across the sidewalk between the playground and a park building. The fault then continues on to Lake Temescal, a former sag pond that was enlarged to form the lake in 1867—just a year before the fault ruptured in the 1868 earthquake. The easiest way to reach Temescal Park is to take the Broadway Terrace exit from northbound California 13. Taking a left on Broadway Terrace, drive under the highway and reach the entrance to the park on the right in less than 100 feet.

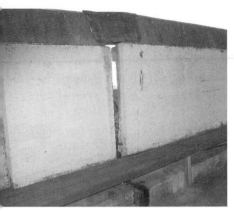

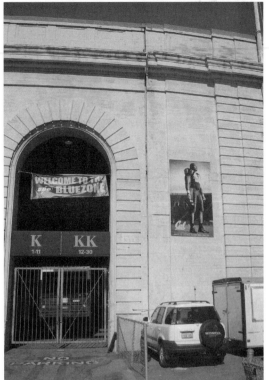

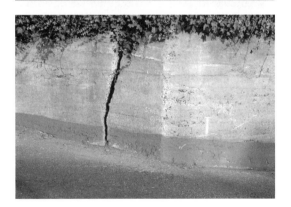

left: Near the southern end of
morial Stadium on the U.C. Berkeley
mpus, creep on the Hayward fault has
it the stadium wall along its entire
tical extent. —RICK MCKENZIE PHOTO

right: Close-up view of the top
ide wall of Memorial Stadium
ICK MCKENZIE PHOTO

tom right: Across the street from the
uth end of Memorial Stadium, creep on
Hayward fault has split and offset a
ncrete retaining wall. (The wall is about
o 8 feet tall at the bottom of the ivy
d about 15 feet tall altogether.)
7 52.19N 122 15.00W)

Another infamous stop on the Hayward fault tour is along the eastern edge of the city of Berkeley. Southeast of the Berkeley campus, the fault manifests itself as the typically abrupt slope break we've seen elsewhere. The elegant Claremont Hotel is yet another grand hotel to achieve a commanding vista and presence by virtue of being located directly atop a fault scarp.

The fault makes an inauspicious entrance into the Berkeley campus, bisecting the university's Memorial Stadium—very nearly through both goalposts. The fault has been a benefactor of generations of Cal students: immediately northeast of the stadium the fault has helped create a little hill, locally known as Cheapskate

Hill for the free view of football games it affords. The fault has been less kind to the stadium itself, taking its inexorable toll as the western half of the stadium moves north with respect to the eastern half. The fault has been equally unkind to walls and other structures adjacent to the stadium.

In the early twentieth century Andrew Lawson (of Lawson Report fame) was a professor of geology at the university. In 1908, he presented an accurate map of the fault, drawing a parallel between its features and those of the San Andreas fault. Nevertheless, fourteen years later, the university drafted the site plan for the stadium. And many decades later, the now-historic structure continues to pose a daunting engineering challenge.

We can find ample evidence of the fault in the natural morphology of the region as well, most notably in the sharp offset of Strawberry Creek, which flows down from the hills and continues through the campus.

Continuing northward from Berkeley, we can find one of the best expressions of the Hayward fault in El Cerrito on the Mira Vista golf course. Although development has obscured many of the subtle fault features in this region, the golf course was established in the early twentieth century and the topographic expression of the fault was preserved.

There, a fault jog creates a sag pond, the sediments of which geologists scrutinized in 1997 to find evidence of prehistoric earthquakes. The 1868 earthquake did not rupture this far north, and there are no historic records of earthquakes on this segment between 1776 and 1868. Given this and the geologic evidence gleaned from the sag pond, researchers think the most recent earthquake struck between about 1640 and 1776. If the fault is trying to slip at 0.3 inch (0.7 centimeters) per year and is unable to move—that is, its locked—it has now stored perhaps 4.5 to more than 6 feet (1.5 to more than 2 meters) of slip—enough to generate an earthquake of at least M6.5. However, there is some debate about the rate of fault creep relative to the rate of overall, long-term slip on the fault. Some scientists have concluded that the level of stored slip on the fault is quite low, which implies an equally low potential for damaging earthquakes. But the issue remains hotly debated.

The earthquake potential of any given fault segment depends not only on its stored slip but also on its length and width. This raises interesting questions when we consider the Hayward fault, ones that we are well-poised to consider now that we have nearly reached the northern terminus of the fault: How long is the Hayward fault? How much of it could rupture at once? Could it rupture along with neighboring faults? The fault leaves land once and for all through a scrubby, undeveloped part of Pinole Park. Toward the south end of the park, we can see the last exposure of the Hayward fault, in the form of a gentle scarp just off of Giant Road, at 37 59.33N 122 21.34W. From here, it is unclear how far the fault continues underwater, or how it connects to faults on the north side of San Pablo Bay.

If the Hayward fault does end at or near San Pablo Bay, we would be left with a couple of possible scenarios for the next large earthquake on the Hayward fault: 1) rupture of the northern segment, from Oakland to San Pablo, which has not produced an earthquake in recorded history; 2) rupture of the northern segment along with all or part of the 1868 segment. Neither of these is particularly comforting to consider given the current population and infrastructure density in the region.

Modern calculations of predicted ground motions from a repeat of the 1868 rupture are sobering, with swaths of heavy damage predicted not only through the East Bay but also around much of the perimeter of the San Francisco Bay on both sides. Even north of San Pablo Bay the predicted ground motions are high enough to cause moderate damage.

But toward the end of the twentieth century, geologists recognized a scenario less comforting still. Geologist David Schwartz and his colleagues investigated the earthquake history of the Rogers Creek fault, which runs from San Pablo Bay northward some 19 to 25 miles (30 to 40 kilometers) before feeding into the Healdsburg fault. Schwartz found evidence of prehistoric earthquakes on the Rogers Creek fault—far bigger events than any that have occurred in recorded history.

As mentioned earlier, by the end of the twentieth century earth scientists had realized that earthquakes do not always respect mapped distinctions between adjacent faults. That is, the Rogers Creek and Healdsburg faults might have been mapped as two separate structures because geologists did not initially judge them to be continuous, but recent earthquakes in other regions suggest that the discontinuity is not large enough to necessarily stop a large rupture that initiates on either fault.

And what, then, of the Rogers Creek fault to the south? By 1999, scientists concluded that they could not rule out a combined Hayward–Rogers Creek rupture. Although they considered it a low probability, such an earthquake could rupture some 60 miles (100 kilometers), not quite on a par with the great earthquakes on the San Andreas fault, but in the same ballpark.

There has always been a bit of rivalry between towns and cities on the San Francisco peninsula and those in the East Bay. San Francisco is San Francisco, whereas Oakland is the "there" that Greer was referring to in her famous quote. But geologically speaking, there is no question that both sides of the bay have substantial faults.

The Calaveras Fault

The Calaveras fault receives less attention than its brother to the west, the Hayward fault. Branching off of the San Andreas fault south of Hollister, the fault bypasses the densely populated central Bay Area. In fact, we might question whether Hollister is fairly part of northern, rather than central, California. Geologically, however, the Calaveras fault is clearly part of the Bay Area fault system. Moreover, extreme land pressures around San Francisco have sent people scrambling farther and farther afield to find affordable homes and business spaces, and the once-sleepy hamlet of Hollister is now considered within the commuting range of the Bay Area. Were a significant earthquake to strike on the Calaveras, a great many buildings and people would lie in its path. However, the Calaveras appears to be creeping over most of its length and may not be able to store enough elastic energy to generate large earthquakes.

No earthquake tour of California would be complete, however, without a stop in Hollister. The once-quiet and fairly rural burg has become far less rural and remote in recent years. For many years, creep along the Calaveras fault took its inexorable toll on Hollister's quaint older homes. Finding faults involved keeping one's eye out for both telltale warping of sidewalks and for houses that looked a little askew. Now, however, the infusion of new—and generally more wealthy—residents has infused the town with a supply of citizens who take their property values seriously. This is good for property upkeep, but less good for the earthquake tourist hoping to find faults.

Nevertheless, the creep rate on the Calaveras fault has been measured at between 0.25 and 0.6 inch (0.7 and 1.5 centimeters) per year since 1910. The

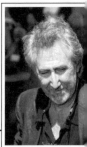

Geologist David Schwartz

David Schwartz: Finding and Connecting the Faults

A geologist who investigates faults using classic geologic techniques as well as paleoseismology, David Schwartz is another scientist whose research interests include some far-flung destinations as well as his own backyard. One of Schwartz's research interests is the nature of the fault systems that bisect the densely populated East Bay region. He concludes that the Hayward fault, which disappears into San Pablo Bay at Pinole, connects with the Rogers Creek fault, which follows a very similar trend northward from the north side of the bay. His work with colleagues at the U.S. Geological Survey and elsewhere further reveals no significant earthquakes on the Rogers Creek fault since at least 1850. The potential for the Hayward fault to generate large earthquakes is a matter of some debate, as it remains unclear if the fault is now creeping enough to prevent the buildup of strain energy. But the Hayward fault has clearly generated damaging earthquakes in the past, and given the likelihood that it is indeed part of a much larger system, the fault represents a substantial hazard to the East Bay area. Work such as Schwartz's illustrates that sometimes the key to hazard assessment is not only to find faults, but to understand how they connect to one another.

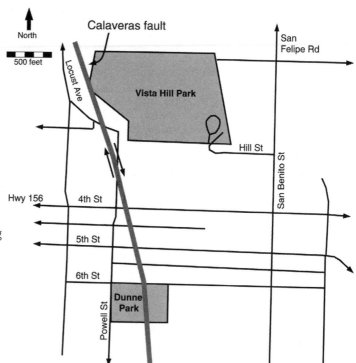

Central Hollister, indicating the trace of the Calaveras fault, which, like the Hayward fault, causes progressive offsets in sidewalks and roads (and damage to houses) as the fault continues to creep.

best intentions of its residents notwithstanding, it is still entirely possible to find faults in Hollister.

The famous walking tour of Hollister begins at the corner of Locust Avenue and Powell Street, near the southwest corner of Vista Hill Park just a few blocks south of Highway 25.

Vista Hill Park, which overlooks central Hollister, is being pushed upward by compression across a small bend in the trace of the Calaveras fault. We can reach the top of the hill by driving west up Hill Street (between 2nd and 3rd Streets) off of San Benito Street, to Vista Hill Park atop the hill, the southwest corner of which is a baseball field. From the edge of the field, we can look down the hill to the picturesque town below, with its quaint older homes and white steepled church. The fault passes along the hill near the base, angling into the town at the corner of Locust Avenue and Powell Street.

To appreciate the features the fault causes as it cuts through Hollister, we can return down the hill and park near Locust and Powell. The fault cuts through this intersection, a characteristic warping of curbs visible in its northeast corner. From here, the fault runs at a slight angle along Locust Street, its trace falling neatly between the house and porch of the home at 359 Locust Street. The fault has largely spared this house, as the fault does not run underneath the primary structure. Decades of steady creep, however, have caused a subtle but noticeable

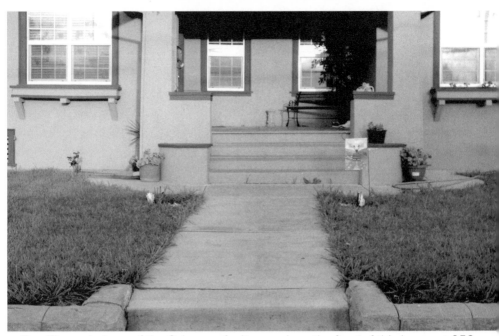

Top: The main trace of the Calaveras fault runs along the front of this house at 359 Locust Street in Hollister. Steady creep on the fault has shifted the front walk, which no longer leads to the center of the porch steps. (36 51.19N 121 24.45W)

Bottom: The creeping Calaveras fault passes between two backyards along this street just north of Dunne Park in Hollister, resulting in progressive southward motion of the house on the right side of the photo. (36 51.03N 121 24.39W)

misalignment between the front porch and the front walk.

Continuing southward on Locust, we follow a more southerly course than the fault, which angles away from the street toward the east. As we cross the successive numbered cross streets, we must look a little farther down each block to find the fault. It is there on almost every block, notwithstanding the best efforts of homeowners to keep their neighborhoods tidy and their homes in one piece.

The final stop on the Hollister tour is on 6th Street just east of Powell Street, at the edge of Dunne Memorial Park.

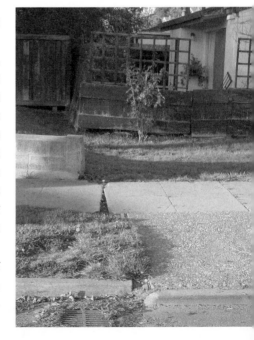

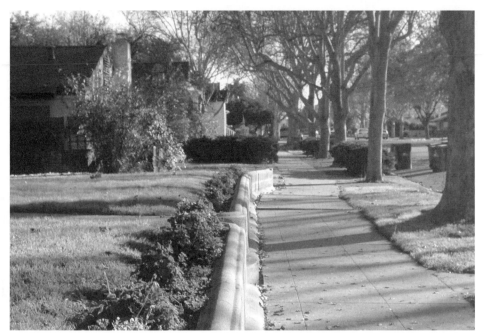

Top: Warping of the low concrete wall in front of the house immediately west of the house shown in the previous photograph (36 51.03N 121 24.39W)

Bottom: The same low concrete wall from the other direction, showing the clear offset in the sidewalk

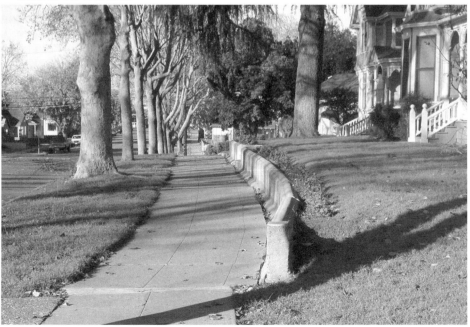

Here again, decades of fault creep have warped the sidewalk and the low walls adjacent to it. The fault trace cuts between two adjacent pieces of property on 6th Street, warping the fence and the curb in front of one of the houses. In time, the property on the east side of the fault will migrate clear into the middle of the road. By this point, the consequences of having a town atop a creeping fault will present a nontrivial challenge for city planners. The view across 6th Street is interesting for another reason: standing at one end and looking down the street across the fault, we can clearly see that the fault moves not along a narrow line but instead over a swath of some width. Such extended fault width is not uncommon. Even if a fault zone is narrow at depth it will commonly cause a zone of more distributed deformation in the loose rock and sediments near the earth's surface.

In Dunne Park itself, no manmade features serve as creep meters, but the fault's handiwork is manifest in a subtle vertical offset that runs north-south through the middle of the park. A similar offset may well have existed at one time elsewhere in Hollister before being smoothed over for property development.

If we follow the trace of the Calaveras fault farther south still, signs of creep become increasingly hard to find. The fault itself largely fades away below Hollister, merging into the creeping San Andreas fault at this juncture. Turning back to view the Calaveras fault from the vantage point of the San Andreas, we can consider the interplay between the San Andreas and the East Bay faults. South of Hollister, the San Andreas fault creeps; north of this juncture the fault is locked. The relative plate motion taken up on the creeping section essentially bifurcates once it reaches the splay of branches, with some motion feeding into creep on the Calaveras fault and some feeding into the locked segment of the San Andreas to the north.

The Northern Plate-Boundary System

In the previous chapter, we explored how the Big Bend controls most of the plate boundary complexity in southern California. In northern California, however, the San Andreas fault is generally simple, and its orientation deviates from the direction of plate motion by a scant 6 degrees, on average. The creeping section may, in fact, creep because there are no geometrical complexities to cause the fault to lock. Along the central part of this segment, the fault creeps at approximately an inch and a half (3 centimeters) per year, taking up most of the total motion of the plates.

But if the middle segment of the San Andreas fault is a singularly straight and uncomplicated tree trunk, how do we account for the explosion of branches that meander through the greater San Francisco Bay Area and continue northward through the less-populated northern coast ranges. This is a good question, and one for which there is no easy answer. Seismologist Mousumi Roy has generated complex numerical/computer models of the fault. Her models show that if the plate boundary beneath the brittle part of the crust is a simple planar offset, then fault branching through the crust might be a natural mechanical consequence of the system. Roy's results are most intriguing, although the question remains: Why here and not elsewhere?

Earth science would be a boring field if we knew the answer to every question. The behavior and evolution of fault systems remains one of the more lively and challenging subfields of both geology and geophysics. This situation is unlikely to change anytime soon, as fault systems are now recognized to fall under a general category of physical processes known as systems science. That is, faults inevitably represent a system whose behavior is extraordinarily complex—one that cannot be understood without integrated and coordinated multidisciplinary investigations. It will, therefore, probably be many years before scientists fully understand the web of faults that represents the plate boundary through northern California. It is clear, however, that these faults represent a system in which the earthquake cycle is a richly and vexingly complex and seemingly inscrutable dance—one whose choreography is, in northern California as elsewhere, both lovely to behold and terrifying to consider.

5 Finding Fault in Central California

Tectonically speaking, the Transverse Ranges define the northern perimeter of southern California. Modern studies of crustal deformation suggest that these mountains behave as a coherent block, with little active faulting—and few earthquakes—currently occurring within the range. Heading northward over the mountains, then, we leave the action behind as soon as we cross thrust faults such as the Sierra Madre at the base of the range's southern front.

The geologic demilitarized zone ends as abruptly as it begins, however, at none other than the San Andreas fault. The San Andreas skirts the northern flank of the mountains from Cajon Pass (north of San Bernardino) to Palmdale and beyond. The segment from Cajon Pass to Tejon Pass, near Palmdale, is known as the Mojave segment, and so this part of the tour perhaps belongs in the following chapter, Finding Fault in the Desert. Geologically, however, it makes sense to parse the San Andreas somewhat differently, as the Mojave segment ruptured with the segment north of Tejon Pass in the 1857 earthquake. Allowing the discussion to follow the great earthquakes, the Mojave segment falls in this chapter. This part of our fault-finding tour will trace the San Andreas over the length of the 1857 rupture, then the creeping zone, and end at the southern terminus of the 1906 rupture in San Juan Bautista.

From the greater Los Angeles region, three primary routes traverse the mountains to intersect the San Andreas fault—and beyond it, central California. The easternmost point of interception is on I-15 north of San Bernardino. The fault crosses I-15 approximately 4 miles north of the I-15/I-215 merge. There the fault zone creates Lone Pine Canyon, a gentle valley that heads northwest away from the freeway. Continuing on I-15, we soon reach the Mojave Desert, where we'll venture in chapter 6. To follow the fault, we exit the freeway at California 138

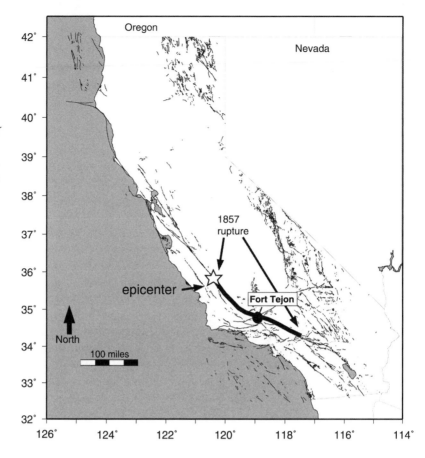

alifornia's major
ults, including
ie San Andreas.
he extent of the
857 rupture is
idicated.

and continue just over a mile to Lone Pine Canyon Road. To reach this intersection, we have to travel a few miles north of the fault. To rejoin the fault, turn
south on Lone Pine Canyon Road and continue about another 1.5 miles until
the road makes a pronounced bend toward the west. From this bend onward,
the road runs through the heart of Lone Pine Canyon, another passageway through
the mountains that eons of motion on the San Andreas fault created.

Lone Pine Canyon is a gift to southland skiers. It leads directly to the mountain communities of Wrightwood and Big Pines and some of the best downhill
skiing close to the greater Los Angeles area. The road has been a bounty for
geologists as well, as it leads directly to sites that have produced some of the
most important information yet gleaned about the history and prehistory of the
San Andreas fault.

With its thick Coulter pines, charming cabin-style homes, and alpine setting,
Wrightwood looks like it belongs in the northern Sierra Nevada—not in mountains a stone's throw away from the megacities of southern California. Its seismic
hazard, however, is inexorably defined by the San Andreas fault, which runs through
the heart of the town. Wrightwood, strewn out along California 2, lies essentially
within the fault zone.

Geologists Tom Fumal, Ray Weldon, and others have focused ongoing paleoseismological studies on Wrightwood. Paleoseismic investigations there have yielded one of the longest records of earthquake prehistory yet determined at any point on the fault. The studies include evidence of at least fourteen earthquakes between A.D. 500 and the present. The last two earthquakes at Wrightwood, in 1812 and 1857, are known historic events.

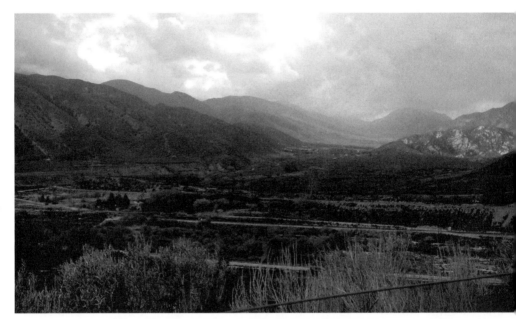

From I-15 north of San Bernardino, the San Andreas fault follows Lone Pine Canyon toward the northwest away from the interstate. (34 15.95N, 117 26.98W)

Traces of ruptures on the San Andreas fault are identified in sedimentary layers in the town of Wrightwood. More recent ruptures extend progressively farther toward the surface, into younger layers. Inferred dates of ruptures are also shown. The two most recent events, in 1812 and 1857, are known historic earthquakes on the San Andreas fault. The others

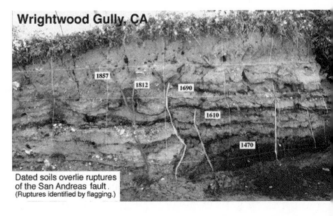

are carbon-14 dates. The string grid, which by established convention forms rectangles 1 meter (roughly 39 inches) long and 1 meter tall, indicates the scale of the photograph.
—TOM FUMAL PHOTO

Ray Weldon: Quantifying the Uncertainties

The San Andreas is arguably both the most famous and the best-studied fault in the world. A small but determined group of geologists has conducted paleoseismic investigations at a number of key sites along the fault to establish the record of prehistoric earthquakes on the San Andreas. The fieldwork itself requires years of painstaking effort. And once completed, paleoseismology provides only snapshots of earthquake records at a small handful of points along the fault. Given the uncertainties of carbon-14 data, which researchers use to establish the dates of earthquakes, it can be difficult—if not impossible—to link the record from one site to another. One of Ray Weldon's interests over the years has been to explore the way paleoseismic results might fit together. In many cases, researchers arrive at ambiguities that cannot be resolved. For example, identified earthquakes with similar dates at different locations could be a single event, or they could be two different earthquakes separated by anywhere from minutes to a few decades. But recognizing ambiguous results is in itself important, as it prevents over-interpretation.

Continuing on California 2 (Big Pines Highway) from Wrightwood to Big Pines, we continue to follow the trace of the San Andreas. The fault is clearly visible as we approach the Big Pines Ranger Station just east of the Mountain High Ski Area in Big Pines. The ranger station sits squarely on top of the fault trace, which runs along the base of the small hill and then continues to the east away from the building.

Just a few hundred yards north of Mountain High, geologists have found evidence of disrupted growth in a small handful of pine trees. Some of the trees have been topped, broken off near the top at some point in the past. Although forces other than earthquakes have topped some trees in this area, in some cases scientists have tied the growth disruption to the timing of the 1857 earthquake. That the rupture dramatically affected trees is not surprising, as anecdotal accounts of the temblor describe trees shaken violently enough to break in two.

Away from Mountain High, Big Pines Highway follows along the fault trace; along some stretches, the road lies within the fault zone. Near Apple Tree Campground 0.9 mile northwest of Big Pines, we come across an exposure of rock south of the road. Once as hard as granite, this rock has been ground to smithereens within the fault zone by innumerable earthquakes over the ages. The powdery consistency of rock at this site illustrates why major fault zones commonly experience more weathering than the surrounding rock.

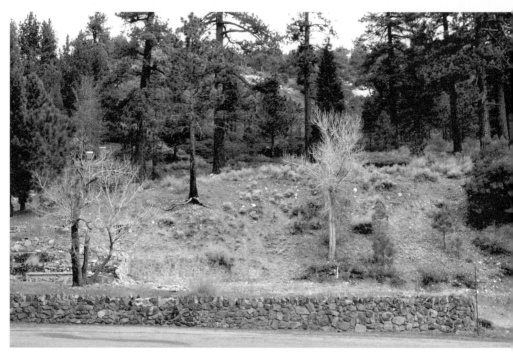

Near Big Pines, the San Andreas fault creates a prominent scarp just north of Big Pines Highway (California 2) and just east of the Big Pines Ranger Station.

To follow the San Andreas away from the Big Pines area, continue on Big Pines Highway toward Palmdale. Once again, the road follows the trace of the San Andreas and the valley the fault has carved in the side of the mountains. Away from Big Pines, the road and the fault descend toward the desert below.

Approximately 3 miles beyond Big Pines, we arrive at Jackson Lake, a lovely, tree-fringed mountain lake popular with anglers and picnickers. Like so many bodies of water along the San Andreas, the elongated shape of Jackson Lake follows the fault trace. In this case, continued fault motion created a so-called shutter ridge, which forms when lateral motion on a fault brings relatively higher ground alongside relatively lower ground. (Imagine a strike-slip fault running through the middle of a small hill. Repeated earthquakes essentially split the hill apart, creating vertical offsets at points along the fault even though the motion has been purely horizontal.) Water filled in the depression nestled behind the ridge to form a lake.

For about 7 miles beyond Jackson Lake, the topography along the road is more complex than we would find along a garden-variety mountain road. Over the ages, the fault has rearranged the landscape in some creative ways. About 12 miles below Big Pines, we arrive at the intersection of Valyermo Road to the west and Bob's Gap Road to the north. Here the fault creates a conspicuous scarp most clearly visible on the northeast corner of the intersection. A small house is perched squarely atop this small hill, poised for a bird's-eye view of the next great southern San Andreas fault earthquake. (It is also poised to fare very poorly in the next earthquake, judging from the fate of houses perched on similar fault-generated ridges during the 1992 Landers earthquake.)

Turning left onto Valyermo Road, we continue downhill, passing a sign for Saint Andrew's Abbey, a small Benedictine monastery with no apparent connection to the San Andreas fault. Turn left onto Pallett Creek Road shortly after passing the abbey and continue another 1.4 miles west to a row of trees south of the road, following a creek bed. This is Pallett Creek, famous in earth-science circles for having been the site of some of the very first paleoseismological investigations. Although at first glance the overall dogleg shape of the creek suggests substantial cumulative offset of the fault, detailed geologic studies reveal that other factors control this bend, and that it is therefore coincidental. Before 1910, the water table was high, and this area was a marshland. The marshland provided layers of peat that are critical to establishing dates of prehistoric earthquakes. An incision of the channel around 1910 drained the swamp, leaving it accessible to paleoseismic investigation. The fault trace cuts diagonally across the creek, causing successive disruption of the marsh sediments within the creek zone. In 1975, then-graduate student Kerry Sieh was the first to excavate these sediments. This was the first in a long series of investigations that eventually yielded a record

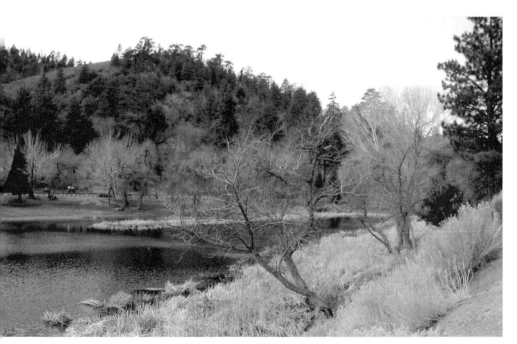

Along the San Andreas fault in the mountains west of Wrightwood, picturesque Jackson Lake owes its existence to the fault. A typical fault-bounded lake, it is thin and long, its length oriented along the fault.

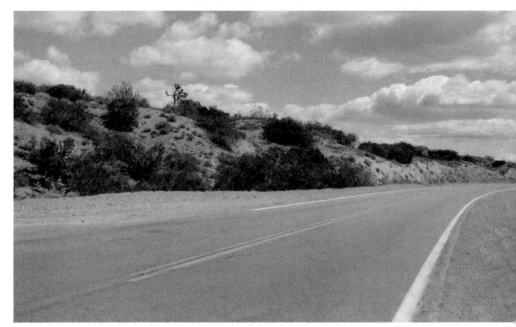

The San Andreas fault creates a low scarp near 47th Street in Palmdale.

of at least nine earthquakes along the fault at this location. The "discovery" of earlier earthquakes agreed with geologist Robert Wallace's earlier conclusion. Wallace analyzed tree rings and found evidence, albeit with only weak age constraints of disrupted growth patterns.

Inspired by earlier trenching studies (by both academic and consulting geologists) that had helped to locate fault traces and investigate prehistoric earthquakes on other faults, Sieh reasoned that the sediments at Pallett Creek might reveal evidence of past earthquakes on the San Andreas fault. Although Sieh's graduate advisors at Stanford gave the idea a mixed reception, Sieh eventually received enough encouragement to launch his first investigations at Pallett Creek. That work eventually extended the known earthquake history from a mere 200 years to more than 1,500 years. The achievement is impressive to consider: from a heap of marshy sediments in an out-of-the-way location, Sieh teased out a chronology dating back to the Dark Ages.

From Pallett Creek, the best way to follow the fault is to proceed along Pallett Creek Road for another 0.8 mile and then turn north (right) onto Longview Road, which veers away from the fault. After another 0.8 mile, we arrive at the intersection with Fort Tejon Road. Turn west (left) on Fort Tejon Road and continue another 2.9 miles to the intersection of 106th Street. This juncture lies north of the San Andreas fault, which runs along the base of the low hill visible to the south. A short drive up 106th Street provides a nice view of the fault zone at the base of the mountains.

Continuing along Fort Tejon Road for another 1.9 miles beyond 106th Street, we arrive at Mount Emma Road. Turn west (left) on Mount Emma Road to rejoin the San Andreas fault in 2.3 miles, although in this area the fault trace is unremarkable. If we continue on to Cheseboro Road and turn right, we soon arrive at Barrel Springs Road, which follows the trace of the fault. From the intersection of Cheseboro and Barrel Springs Roads until we reach 47th Street, the fault scarp is just north of the road at the base of a low hill. At the intersection with 40th Street, the fault crosses the road; cottonwood trees on the south side of the road delineate the trace of the fault.

Continuing along the next 3.3 miles (along a sharp bend at which the road becomes 25th Street), we pass a lovely development of new housing—all within spitting distance of the San Andreas fault. We are again reminded that the 50-foot no-man's land dictated by the Alquist-Priolo Act (and discussed in chapter 2) is sometimes not very wide, given the scale of major fault zones—not to mention the hazard they pose. (The act stipulates a no-build zone around each active strand within a fault zone; in some areas the total width is greater than 50 feet.) After 3.3 miles, turn left (west) on Avenue S to head toward California 14.

Approaching California 14 on Avenue S, the fault is on our left. In this area, the fault scarp forms a linear ridge, the continuation of which forms the northern edge of Lake Palmdale. The Lamont Odett Vista Point off of California 14 northbound, just south of the Avenue S exit, offers a good perspective of the lake and the fault scarp.

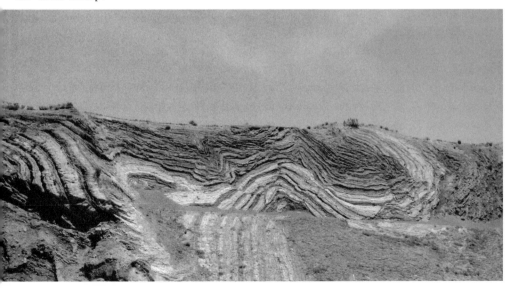

Arguably the most famous roadcut in the world, this site just north of Lake Palmdale provides a spectacular exposure not of the San Andreas fault itself but of how dramatic forces can shape rocks immediately adjacent to a major fault zone. The fault itself runs just south of the hill containing the roadcut. (34 33.76N 118 07.99W)

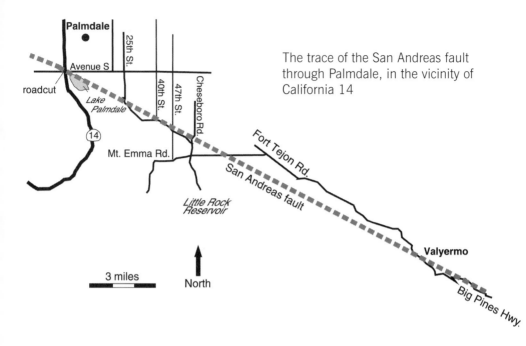

The trace of the San Andreas fault through Palmdale, in the vicinity of California 14

Probably the best known point of interception with the San Andreas fault north of Los Angeles is associated with this scarp, and we can find it in a roadcut on California 14 just a stone's throw from Lake Palmdale. Here motion on the fault has bent and folded rocks in improbable ways. This deformation is exhibited spectacularly in a roadcut just north of Lake Palmdale, arguably the most famous roadcut in the world. The twisted rocks do not represent the fault itself but rather continued motion on and squeezing across the fault zone. Stopping along California 14 is neither legal nor safe, but we can enjoy a double view of the amazing roadcut by taking the following exit to the north (Palmdale Boulevard) and doubling back along the freeway. We can also exit the highway at Avenue S and walk up the small hill on the west side of the road to enjoy a safe view of the fault's exquisite handiwork.

Although our fault tour has proceeded from Cajon Pass toward Tejon Pass, we can see a number of interesting fault features by taking California 14 directly from the San Fernando Valley to Palmdale and taking a short 10-mile detour away from the highway. Although the drive to or from Wrightwood offers spectacular scenery as well as geology, we do not have to venture too far off the beaten track to find faults near Palmdale.

Away from California 14, the San Andreas fault creates a gentle valley that heads northwest away from the highway and continues on to cross I-5 near the small town of Gorman. State Road N2 follows along this trace of the fault. The intersection of N2 and California 14 is a few miles north of the fault, but N2 heads nearly due west and rejoins the fault zone in a few short miles. Along N2, we can find numerous fault features, including Lake Elizabeth and Lake Hughes, two more slivers of lakes nestled within depressions the fault created.

We can reach the next interesting fault juncture, the intersection of the fault with I-5, by either continuing from the east or, more directly, via I-5 from Los Angeles. Whereas many of the fault tours discussed in this book follow rarely driven roads, such as N2, the heavily trafficked I-5 provides a good fault-finding opportunity for the accidental earthquake tourist. Approaching the exit signs for Gorman off of I-5, the highway makes a pronounced bend to the left as it joins the valley. On Gorman Post Road, just east and south of the freeway exit, we find a convenient (and safe) vantage point from which to view the valley and the path of the San Andreas fault.

Continuing farther along I-5, we soon arrive at Fort Tejon, which lent its name to the 1857 earthquake. Fort Tejon itself was a somewhat less auspicious namesake. According to an account published in a San Francisco newspaper in 1863, Lt. Francisco Ruiz first bestowed the name Cañada del Tejon—Badger Canyon— on the canyon in 1803, after a dead badger was found at the entrance to the canyon.

Established in 1854 to "control" Native American populations in the region, Fort Tejon was occupied by the U.S. Army for a scant single decade, and its two primary claims to fame could scarcely be more disparate. First, it gave rise to

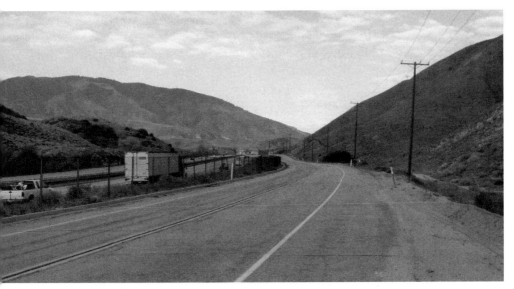

At the small town of Gorman, the San Andreas fault creates a northwest-trending valley that I-5 follows. The photo was taken alongside Gorman Post Road, which parallels I-5 here. (34 47.60N 118 50.20W)

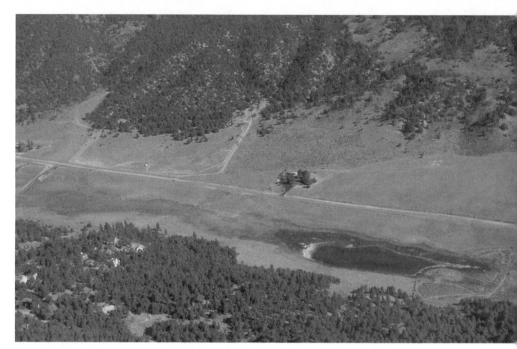

The San Andreas fault creates a small linear valley and sag pond near Frazier Park, just west of the town of Gorman. From I-5 near Gorman, Cuddy Canyon Road follows the fault zone toward the west-northwest. —SUSAN HOUGH PHOTO; PILOTING BY BILL MURRELL

the legend of the U.S. Camel Corps, a saga that found its way into some fairly respectable history books in spite of being (so to speak) quite the tall tale. Camels were kept at the fort for a few months in late 1859 and early 1860, but only until they could be auctioned off. These animals were temporarily served by their country at Fort Tejon, not vice versa.

Fort Tejon's second claim to fame stemmed from its existence at the time of the great earthquake that would become the fort's namesake. Traditionally, scientists name earthquakes for the city or town—occasionally the geographic feature—closest to the epicenter of the event. Occasionally, the naming of modern earthquakes becomes controversial when people in neighboring towns resent either having been "stuck with" an earthquake or, just as often, not having been duly recognized as the focal point of damage. However, people of European descent were few and far between in southern California at the time, so Fort Tejon had little competition in 1857. (To my knowledge, no name of Native American origin was bestowed on an earthquake in the United States until the 2001 Nisqually earthquake near Seattle.)

In any case, Fort Tejon exists today as a historic landmark, just a few miles north of where the fault crosses I-5 at Gorman. To follow the San Andreas fault

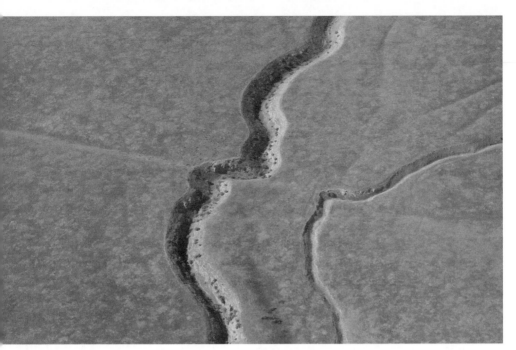

A bird's-eye view of the San Andreas fault in the Carrizo Plain. The fault creates the subtle linear grove that runs diagonally across the photograph. Two stream channels have been offset in a right-lateral sense by large earthquakes, including the 1857 Fort Tejon event. —SUSAN HOUGH PHOTO; PILOTING BY BILL MURRELL

as it heads away from Gorman, we must again head into terrain that quickly becomes mountainous and fairly remote as the fault once again leaves the desert floor to enter more mountainous terrain. From I-5, Frazier Mountain Peak Road leads to Cuddy Valley Road, a route that offers some lovely sites for camping and hiking on and near Frazier Mountain. The San Andreas fault runs through—and has created—a series of valleys along this route: Leona Valley, Cuddy Valley, and Pine Canyon. We can find typical fault features along these valleys and canyons, including a classic sag pond along the fault in Cuddy Valley.

Away from the Frazier Mountain area, the fault enters terrain that is more remote still and becomes difficult to follow. In the greater scheme of things, of course, it is not a bad thing to keep one's faults in remote regions, where their ability to cause mischief will be reduced. Certainly, however, more than enough real estate and lives are in proximity to the San Andreas between Cajon and Tejon Passes. A repeat of the 1857 rupture would generate not only severe shaking in nearby desert communities such as Palmdale, but also potentially damaging ground motion throughout much of the greater Los Angeles and San Bernardino regions.

The 1857 rupture continued well northward of Fort Tejon, too, but without a private plane at our disposal, we earthquake tourists will find it difficult to follow the fault as it bends to a more northerly direction west of Tejon Pass.

Our tour of the San Andreas fault through central California will therefore embark on a brief detour. Continuing northward on I-5, we enter the Central Valley, a corridor of the state better known for zippy highway speeds than scenery of any stripe—cultural or geological.

At first, the vast, flat expanse of the valley might evoke thoughts of Kansas more than of California; its geology appears to be only marginally less featureless and enduring. This stability appears to be no illusion, at least on a local scale. Researchers have used years of GPS data to map out the so-called velocity field within southern California. Such results reveal the slow accrual of strain building in the crust. And at least over recent times, the Central Valley appears to be another region that is moving as a coherent block, with little or no strain building on any faults within its perimeter. For reasons not entirely understood, overall plate motion is taken up by the San Andreas fault, offshore faults, and fault systems that run through the Mojave Desert, north through the Owens Valley, and beyond. The Central Valley, thus, appears to be a coherent parcel of flotsam sandwiched between the state's active earthquake zones.

To rejoin the San Andreas from I-5, California 58 provides a convenient route of passage. Leaving the interstate at this exit, we pass through an impressive strip of GFL (gas, food, lodging) establishments. This is not a bad place to stop and refuel, as such way stations become few and far between as we head west away from the interstate.

Following California 58 away from I-5, we pass through a land that time seems to have forgotten. This part of the

Don Argus:
Finding Fault from Space

One of the relatively new items in the fault-finding scientist's bag of tricks is the Global Positioning System (GPS). By recording signals from GPS satellites in orbit around the earth, scientists can track positions on land with high accuracy. In recent years, such techniques have allowed us to watch the plates move. Scientists such as Don Argus at the Jet Propulsion Laboratory in Pasadena have also used GPS data to figure out where strain is building in the crust. Where we can identify a strain signal, we can also infer the fault, or faults, on which it is building. Recalling the cartoon illustrating elastic-rebound theory (see page 10), such measurements help scientists identify where curved lines are forming in the neighborhood of a locked fault. GPS is generally the domain of a branch of science known as geodesy: the study of the shape of the earth's surface. But whereas classic geodesy generally views the shape of the earth as static, Don Argus and other modern geodesists are exploiting the newest tools of the trade to investigate how the shape changes—in some cases, finding faults.

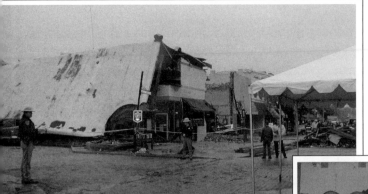

Shaking from the December 2003 San Simeon earthquake collapsed the roof of this historic masonry building in downtown Paso Robles, killing two people.
—RAKESH K. GOEL PHOTO

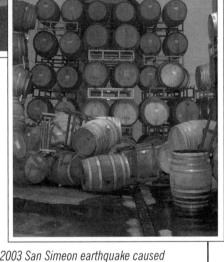

The 2003 San Simeon earthquake caused nonstructural damage to several wineries in the Paso Robles area, including these toppled wine barrels at the Turley Vineyards in the city of Templeton. —PATRICIA GROSSI PHOTO, COURTESY OF RISK MANAGEMENT SOLUTIONS, INC.

The Quake that Stopped the Presses

This chapter is devoted to a tour of the San Andreas fault, the most important fault in central California and the one that offers the best fault-finding opportunities in this part of the state. But the earth has a knack of dishing up a serving of humility to earthquake scientists (and writers) who take the planet's complexity too lightly. I found myself suitably chastened on the morning of December 22, 2003, when an earthquake struck west of the San Andreas fault, on one of the many thrust faults in the San Simeon–Paso Robles area—a part of California I had not discussed in this book! The San Simeon earthquake did not generate a dramatic surface rupture; early indications are that the rupture did not reach the surface at all. Fault-finding opportunities in this part of the state thus remain limited.

Although temblors are relatively infrequent in this part of the state, earthquakes of consequence do strike: the M6.5 quake of 2003 killed two people and caused substantial damage in Paso Robles and nearby communities. Half a century earlier, on November 22, 1952, a M6.0 temblor had rocked the same area. Fault maps of the area reveal a web of mapped faults, most with a northwest-southeast alignment. Scientists do not expect these faults to generate activity on a par with faults such as the San Andreas or San Jacinto. But the lesson of the 2003 San Simeon quake is clear: California—*all* of California—is earthquake country.

Central Valley, which includes the quietly and quaintly dusty farming communities of Buttonwillow and McKittrick, is cotton country. Here again the landscape evokes thoughts of a timeless Midwest breadbasket region far more than a dynamic plate-boundary system.

Soon enough, however, the landscape starts to remind the earthquake tourist that he or she is not in Kansas anymore. Following the bends in California 58 away from McKittrick, we arrive at a set of gentle hills. As we press onward and climb away from the valley, the road becomes steeper and more sinuous. Still the grass-covered hills appear gentle, even peaceful. It is worth stopping at one of the scenic vistas along the drive, if only to view the valley below and to listen to the songs of birds and gentle breezes—and very little more. By this time, we have truly reached one of the less-traveled byways in the heart of this bustling and densely populated state.

We should not, however, let the apparent tranquility of the setting fool us. The hills are known as the Temblor Range. Although obviously of Spanish origin, the origins of this name are interesting to consider. Before the twentieth century, the usage appears to have been primarily local, as only the collective term Coast Range appears on maps through at least the late 1800s. But in the vicinity of Wallace Creek, we find references from the mid- to late 1800s to not only the Temblor Range but also the Temblor District and the Temblor House. An interesting question then arises: Were these names bestowed before or after the 1857 earthquake? The notes from an 1855 survey of the region describe the mountains as "Broken Mountains" and "Rough Mountains." Apparently, then, the mountains in the area did not carry the name prior to the Fort Tejon event, which suggests that no substantial seismic activity rocked the region in the years leading up to 1857.

The Temblor Range exists because the alignment of the San Andreas fault does not match perfectly with the direction of plate motion. This gives rise to a small component of compression, or squeezing, that has caused the crust to ripple. This is the same process of squeezing across the fault that creates the Transverse Ranges, but we see it here on a far more modest scale.

The curves along California 58 become more tortuous as we climb farther into the hills. Consider it a sign of things to come.

The descent from the peak of the Temblor Range is steeper than the ascent. At the base of the hills we arrive at a sign for 7 Mile Road, which branches south-southwest away from the highway. A left to the south-southwest on this road leads quickly to a wide, well-graded dirt road on the left. As we turn onto this road and proceed south, the Temblor Range and the San Andreas fault are to our left. One of the best places in the state—if not on earth—to find evidence of active strike-slip faulting lies 4.1 miles south of the turn from 7 Mile Road. Continuing along through the apparent middle of nowhere, we pass a couple of of aging hulks of vehicles that seem to be eroding back to dust on a geologic time scale. A sign and a small wooden parking corral mark our destination: the Wallace Creek Interpretive Trail.

Constructed by the Bureau of Land Management with input from SCEC scientists and personnel, the trail heads east from the parking lot toward the base of the hills. A sign at the trailhead is usually well stocked with trail guides; you can also find them on the Web.

As we walk along the trail, the hills look subdued and unremarkable—the kind of topographic undulation common throughout much of California. A sign at the base of the hills provides information about the fault, but the best vantage point for finding the fault lies at the top of a short, steep trail up the hills. Climbing and looking down to the northwest, we find a dramatic slash of Zorro in the landscape. This is Wallace Creek.

The man for whom Wallace Creek was named, geologist Robert Wallace, was one of the first geologists to explore this stretch of the fault in detail. Wallace Creek is one of the most dramatic and best-studied examples of an offset stream channel to be found anywhere along the San Andreas fault. The creek is but one of a steady progression of streams that flow down the western flank of the Temblor

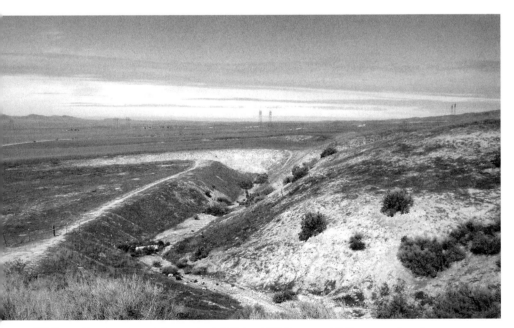

Wallace Creek, named for geologist Robert Wallace, exhibits a spectacular Z-shaped offset where it crosses the San Andreas fault. Detailed investigations at this site have provided some of the best estimates of the long-term slip rate of the fault. (35 16.26N 119 49.60W)

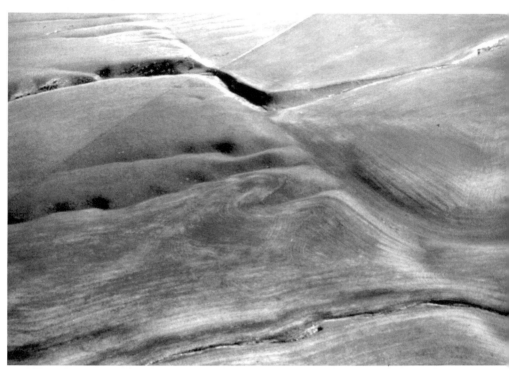

We can best appreciate the handiwork of the San Andreas fault from the air. From this vantage point, the offset of drainages—including the largest and most conspicuous, Wallace Creek—is clear. —BOB WALLACE PHOTO

Range, the best view of which is from the air. Such features are common along the San Andreas, but here the fault trace is relatively simple and narrow, and so the offset channels are displayed to dramatic effect.

By dating organic material within the streambed of Wallace Creek, Kerry Sieh estimated that approximately 3,800 years have elapsed since the creek cut straight down the hill. In that time, the fault has offset the creek by a total of approximately 140 yards. The overall slip rate along the fault, then, has been approximately 1.3 inches (3.4 centimeters) per year. Because this section of the fault remains stubbornly locked, the motion does not accrue steadily but rather piecemeal, and in dramatic fashion. Scientists estimate that the 1857 Fort Tejon earthquake offset Wallace Creek by a whopping 11 yards (10 meters). Assuming this was a typical amount of slip for great earthquakes on this segment, another easy calculation reveals that perhaps thirteen or fourteen earthquakes have struck this segment of the fault in the last 3,800 years; that's a rate of one every 290 years, on average.

As we've already discussed, the Pacific–North American plate-boundary system encompasses nearly the full width of California. But if we want to point to a spot that largely *is* the plate boundary, we can perhaps find no better spot than Wallace Creek.

We cannot see some of the most important features at Wallace Creek, however, because they lie beneath the ground. Since the 1980s, Kerry Sieh, Lisa Grant, Jing Liu, Charlie Rubin, and others have extensively investigated the fault at and near Wallace. Charlie Rubin and his colleagues have additionally investigated a site a few hundred yards south of Wallace Creek. These investigations again involved the digging of long trenches across and next to the fault, trenches in which the sediments reveal evidence of great prehistoric earthquakes. A few miles south of Wallace Creek, at Phelan Ranch, Grant and Sieh assembled evidence for five earthquakes over the past 800 years, or one every 160 years. The discrepancy between this value and the estimate based on long-term offset implies that some ruptures involved less slip than the 11 yards (10 meters) that accompanied the 1857 quake. This, in turn, has interesting implications for the behavior of major faults. It suggests that their earthquakes are not regular in either their timing or their amount of slip.

Walking along the Wallace Creek trail, we find additional evidence of faulting, including other offset stream channels. South of the short trail, the handiwork of the fault is subtle, but we can trace it by eye as it fades into the distance.

The return walk along the trail toward Wallace Creek and then back to the parking lot provides a good opportunity to turn our gaze west, away from the fault and toward the Carrizo Plain.

Kerry Sieh: A Voyage Back in Time

When Kerry Sieh began his paleoseismological work at Pallett Creek, he was still a graduate student at Stanford, and the entire subfield was in its infancy. Most fault studies focused on the investigation of faults through rock, not the dissection of messy, marshy layer cakes whose sediments had been disrupted by prehistoric earthquakes. Working first at Pallett Creek and ultimately with students of his own at other sites, Sieh established the first—and still one of the longest—records of prehistoric earthquakes known from geologic evidence. Paleoseismology is not about finding faults per se, but rather about extending fault studies into the critical fourth dimension: time.

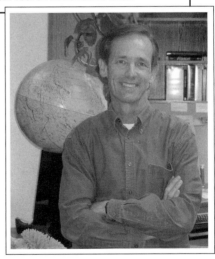

Geologist Kerry Sieh in his office at Caltech

Hundreds of years ago the Carrizo Plain was home to native tribes, including the Chumash and Yokut. Now sparsely populated, the region is home to a sprinkling of hardy human souls as well as

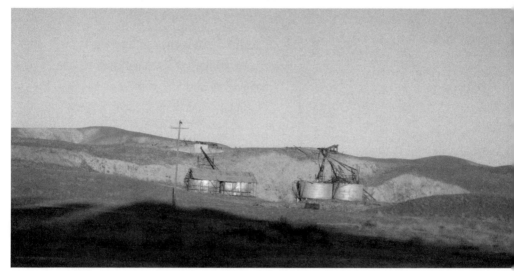

Along Bitterwater Road north of Wallace Creek, the San Andreas fault creates a rift valley. Although the fault zone can be complex and broad in this region, we can see a clear fault scarp at some locations. (35 34.33N 120 07.53W)

a diverse collection of wildlife, including giant kangaroo rats, tule elk, and pronghorns. As of 2001, some 250,000 acres of this unique, pastoral corridor were under the protection and care of the Nature Conservancy.

Returning in the car along the dirt road toward California 58, we follow the fault, the structure of which becomes somewhat more complex and difficult to trace north of Wallace Creek. To follow the fault north beyond California 58, we must again take a brief detour west, away from the fault, as no road continues along the fault. Turning west on California 58, we head into the Carrizo Plain, traversing some sharply rolling hills before reaching Bitterwater Road some 15.4 miles after the junction of California 58 and 7 Mile Road. A two-lane paved road that runs approximately from nowhere to nowhere, Bitterwater Road sees far more ground squirrel cross traffic than through-going automobile traffic. Driving the road at certain times of year, we are reminded of nothing less than a carnival shooting gallery, except that in this case we can only do our best to avoid the multitude of scampering furry critters that dart across our path. Fortunately, these seemingly hapless creatures appear to be expert at darting not only into but also out of the way of oncoming vehicles.

For the first 8.5 miles or so, ground squirrels remain the primary point of interest along Bitterwater Road, but then the road makes a bend to the east, and things start to get interesting. At this point, the road has rejoined the San Andreas fault and the relatively wide valley in which it lies. Here the fault zone is several hundred yards wide; geologists have found evidence for discrete fault traces throughout the width of this zone.

Ramón Arrowsmith:
Understanding the Landscape

Geologist Ramón Arrowsmith has spent years investigating the San Andreas fault in south-central California. He recently extended his work on the San Andreas fault to a similar (but left-lateral) strike-slip fault in northern Tibet—the Altyn Tagh fault. With one of his graduate students, Arrowsmith has obtained some of the first information about the earthquake history along this fault and its role in the collision between the Indian and Eurasian plates.

Back in California, Arrowsmith has worked extensively on the Carrizo and Cholame segments of the San Andreas fault. These segments pass through semiarid grasslands in which fault features tend to remain well preserved over centuries. Among other endeavors, Arrowsmith has focused on the fault's handiwork in shaping topography. The landscape along the fault results from the interplay between the tectonic processes that deform the crust and the surface processes, such as erosion, that sculpt it. By focusing on the detailed nature of scarps, offset stream channels, and other fault-related features, Arrowsmith has not only described the characteristics of the fault zone itself but also contributed to our understanding of the long-term rate of earthquakes along the central San Andreas fault. Although seemingly timeless, the character of the land in this region is in a geologic sense ephemeral: the long-term slip rate on the San Andreas fault is so high—

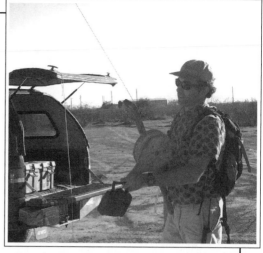

Ramón Arrowsmith has developed a system to photograph faults using a remotely triggered camera flown aloft by a kite or balloon. He has deployed this system to study faults around the world, including in China (top) and closer to home in Arizona (bottom).

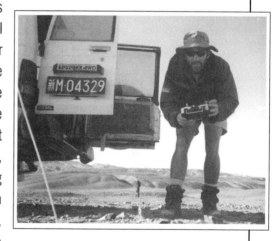

1.4 inches (35 millimeters) per year—that the faulting will completely reorganize the landscape in less than a million years. The pace of change is much different in Arizona, where Arrowsmith now lives, where one typically views landscapes that have been stable for 1 to 2 million years.

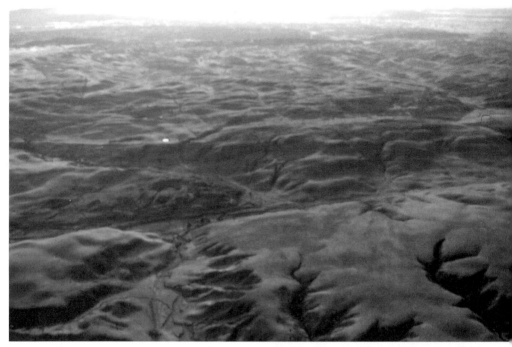

Seen from above, the San Andreas fault cuts across, and shifts, the course of Bitterwater Creek. From the ground it can be difficult to trace individual fault features; from the air their overall alignment is far more obvious. —RAMÓN ARROWSMITH PHOTO

For the most part, the rift valley along Bitterwater Road is broad, gentle, and complex, but linear fault scarps are visible in some areas, including along the low hill east of the road behind one of the few houses along this stretch.

Bitterwater Road veers to the west, away from the rift valley, about 22.3 miles north of California 58, and soon intersects California 46, a busy car and truck route linking I-5 to Paso Robles. At this juncture we are quickly aware that we have left behind the bucolic back roads of California.

Taking California 46 eastward, we soon arrive at the small town of Cholame, where we rejoin the San Andreas fault. Cholame is in San Luis Obispo County, one of the state's original twenty-seven counties and founded in 1850 before the state joined the Union in September of that year. In 1850, San Luis Obispo County had a population of 336 people—rancheros and their employees—strewn out over great ranches that covered a half million acres. Cholame itself was incorporated in 1852.

In recent times Cholame has had two primary claims to fame. First, it was on this stretch of California 46 that James Dean had his fatal two-car accident in 1965. A memorial marks the site of the crash, just east of the Jack Ranch Café.

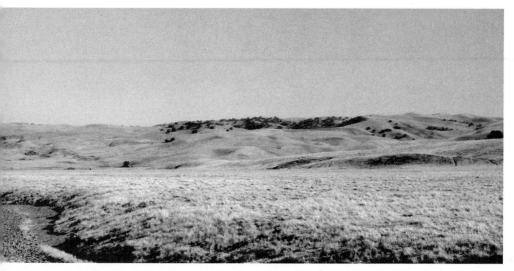

This photo, taken north of California 46 looking south, shows the transition between the creeping section of the San Andreas fault *(foreground)* and the 1857 rupture zone. This segment of the fault broke in 1857, but no clear rupture features are visible. The fault trace runs along the bottom edge of the first set of low hills. (35 45.44N 120 18.40W)

Just south of California 46 along Davis Road, the San Andreas fault creates a prominent scarp that runs southward along the base of low hills. (35 43.49N 120 16.88W)

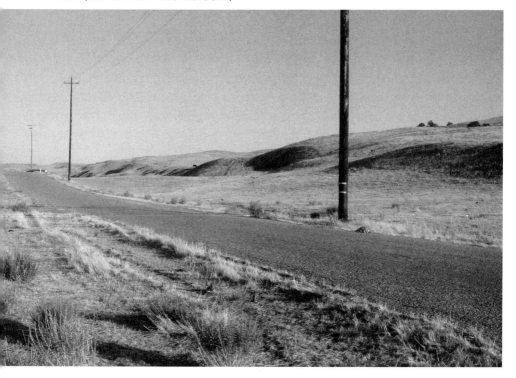

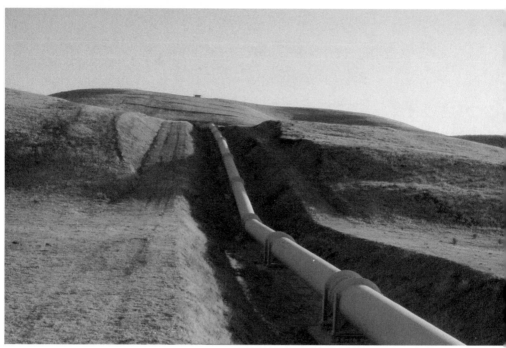

A gas pipe that crosses the trace of the San Andreas fault just south of California 46 near Cholame was built above ground to facilitate repairs following a major earthquake. (35 43.41N 120 16.77W)

Second, and more important for our purposes, Cholame represents an important geologic crossroads for the San Andreas fault. South of Cholame, the fault is locked, slipping only in major earthquakes. Immediately north of California 46, however, the fault behavior begins a transition from locked to creeping. The Cholame segment of the fault is creeping at present, but it ruptured during the 1857 earthquake. The fault, thus, appears to be creeping at a rate that does not account for the full long-term slip rate on the fault. Either that or the behavior of the fault—locked versus creeping—must change over time.

In any case, finding the fault trace along California 46 is complicated by the need to avoid becoming earthquake tourist roadkill. Therefore we turn right (south) on Davis Road, 4.2 miles east of the intersection with Bitterwater Road. The fault crosses Davis Road 0.6 mile south of California 46, beyond which it creates a pronounced scarp to the west of the road. Another 0.3 mile south, we arrive at an interesting sight: just west of the road a large white gas pipe emerges from the ground like a giant worm and traverses a short distance on low supports above ground before disappearing below the surface again. This peculiar arrangement marks the main trace of the fault, and was designed to keep the pipe from being torn apart underground during an earthquake.

Returning to California 46, we turn right (east) and proceed a short 0.1 mile to a left (north) turn lane, which leads to Cholame Road. This road once again more or less follows the fault on its course nearly due north. Just north of California 46, the fault creates a low scarp visible to the west. We can clearly see the scarp as we travel Cholame Road 1.5 to 2 miles north of the highway.

Continuing farther along Cholame Road, we drive along a valley created by the interplay of fault segments. The fault segment to the west of the valley gradually dies out in favor of a segment along the eastern side of the valley. Where the segments overlap, extensional forces have created the valley between them. Eight miles north of California 46, the eastern segment runs along Gold Hill, the low hill to the east of the road.

After 10.4 miles from California 46, we cross a small, nondescript bridge. Just 0.1 mile north of this bridge, a small broken pipe is nestled under a tree just north of the road. This pipe, which we'll discuss later, broke in 1966 some nine hours before the 1966 Parkfield earthquake. Drive beyond the bridge to see

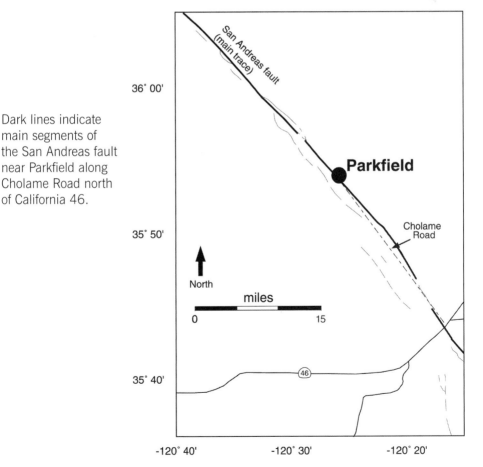

Dark lines indicate main segments of the San Andreas fault near Parkfield along Cholame Road north of California 46.

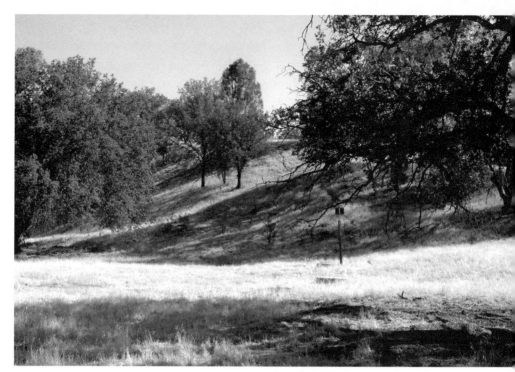

The main trace of the San Andreas fault runs along the base of this hill, a fault scarp, south of the town of Parkfield. The U.S. Geological Survey has installed an instrument at this location to measure fault creep. (35 51.53N 120 23.54W)

The San Andreas fault cuts along the top of a hill on private property just south of the town of Parkfield, creating a gentle, linear valley.

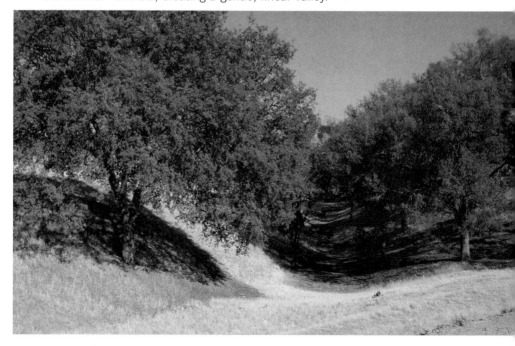

a small scarp that the fault created west of the road. The road bends toward the west about 2 miles beyond the bridge; beyond that point the fault trace continues through hills east of the road, through private property.

About 13 miles from California 46, we arrive at Turkey Flat, a small valley immediately adjacent to the fault. This unassuming glen was the site of a seismological shoot-out of sorts in the late 1980s and early 1990s. Scientists and geotechnical engineers from around the globe were invited to visit the site and use the method of their choice to determine the velocity of seismic shear waves within the sedimentary valley. The project was the brainchild of a group of scientists pulled together by the International Association of Seismology and Physics of the Earth's Interior, known in earth-science circles as IASPEI. Seismologist Brian Tucker took the lead in launching the project. The California Division of Mines and Geology (now the California Geological Survey) provided key data for the experiment. A number of groups supported by a range of different agencies, including some in Japan, made the velocity measures.

Such measurements provide the most critical information for assessing the amplification of waves within any sedimentary basin or valley—a critical factor in overall seismic hazard, as shaking is amplified, sometimes substantially, within near-surface sediments. In general, the "softer" (that is, lower velocity) the sediments, the greater the amplification. But while scientists have developed myriad methods to determine shear-wave velocities in shallow sediments, rarely are the methods tested against one another or against any sort of ground truth.

The Turkey Flat challenge yielded discouraging lessons: velocity estimates vary considerably depending on the method used to determine them, and the uncertainties in velocity measurements translate into significant uncertainties in estimates of amplification. It may be fairly easy to predict effects of sediment-induced amplification in a gross sense, but fairly difficult to predict in fine detail.

Leaving the issue—and Turkey Flat—behind and pressing onward, the road catches up to the fault again about 15.5 miles north of California 46. Here the fault runs beneath a low, white bridge that leads into Parkfield. The 1966 rupture pulled the bridge apart, and repairing it required extending it by several feet. For years, the bridge provided clear clues into the nature of the fault and earthquake, but eventually the bridge was rebuilt with a massive concrete undercarriage from which the earthquake tourist can learn little.

Turning right and crossing the bridge, we arrive at Parkfield, the self-proclaimed Earthquake Capital of the World. Parkfield's proudly embraced heritage stems primarily from having been the site of a series of moderate earthquakes between 1857 and 1966; on average, one every 22.6 years. This apparent regularity led to the so-called Parkfield Prediction Experiment, a major monitoring effort on the part of the U.S. Geological Survey designed to catch the next Parkfield earthquake red-handed. At the time the experiment was launched, researchers expected the next

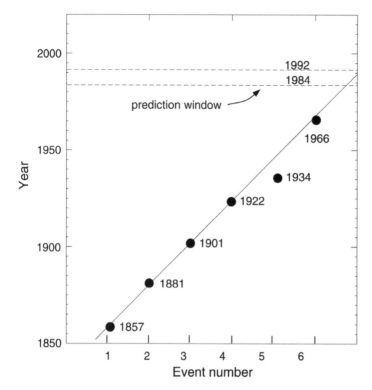

A series of apparently regular historic earthquakes near Parkfield led to the Parkfield Prediction experiment and the specific prediction of an earthquake within four years of 1988.

Parkfield earthquake to strike within four years of 1988. However, seismologists found themselves waiting for Godot—for 14 years and counting after 1988.

The failure of the prediction notwithstanding, monitoring at Parkfield has provided scientists with a bounty of information about the behaviors of earthquakes and faults. Even the failed prediction itself has been a tremendous learning opportunity—not to mention a tremendous lesson in humility. Perhaps most important, Parkfield taught us that a regular series of earthquakes can occur on faults or fault systems whose long-term behavior is quite complex and not nearly as predictable as it may appear.

Parkfield's importance, however, goes far beyond the prediction of moderate earthquakes, because the 1857 Parkfield event was no ordinary M6.0 earthquake. The 1857 event was two earthquakes of about M6.0 that preceded the great 1857 Fort Tejon temblor by a couple of hours. This suggests that Parkfield might be something of a critical preparation zone.

Moreover, several lines of evidence, including the enigmatic observation of a pipe break about nine hours before the 1966 Parkfield earthquake, suggest that Parkfield earthquakes may be preceded by significant creep events. That is, before the earthquakes begin, the fault might experience an episode of creep—slip that is too slow and steady to generate seismic waves. And herein lies a large measure of the scientific interest in Parkfield: if precursory creep events do occur, then we have a fighting chance of catching these events in the act and buying at least a few minutes of warning before a major temblor strikes.

A few minutes might not sound like much, but a lot can be done in a short amount of time if systems are designed properly. Currently, the only viable early warning technology exploits not precursors but rather the difference in the speed of electromagnetic waves and seismic waves. It is essentially the same difference as that between the speed at which lightning and thunder reach our senses, except that seismic waves are basically sound waves that travel through the ground instead of the air. If a seismometer near a fault can sense the initiation of a large earthquake, a signal can be sent, perhaps via microwave communication, to distant locations and arrive ahead of the seismic waves. For such a system to work, large earthquakes must commence some distance from the sites where warnings will be issued; otherwise the warning will be too short to do any good. Returning to the weather analogy, a close earthquake would generate the nearly simultaneous flash-BOOM that occurs when lightning strikes nearby.

Ideal settings for early warning systems exist at a number of places around the globe. These include Mexico City, at risk from coastal subduction-zone earthquakes several hundred miles away, and Japan, whose major cities are also at

Early Warning System

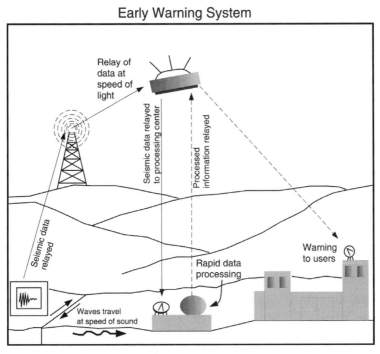

The principle of so-called early warning systems, whereby an electromagnetic signal moving at the speed of light transmits advance notice of strong shaking and arrives at distant sites ahead of the earthquake waves, which travel at the speed of sound.

risk from large offshore earthquakes such as the great 1923 Kanto temblor near Tokyo. Indeed, the oldest successful early warning system in the world is in Japan, where automated systems bring bullet trains to a stop when a significant earthquake strikes.

If precursory creep is common prior to large earthquakes, the prospects for early warning would be vastly improved. A few minutes can be enough time not only to stop trains but also to warn airplanes, to shut down critical systems and computer hard drives, to get people to safe locations inside or outside, and more.

Unfortunately, while the lightning-and-thunder early warning systems are based on well-established physics, the prospects for systems based on precursory creep remain speculative at best. Seismologists need much more research, and data from large earthquakes, to determine if science fiction can become science fact. Parkfield continues to represent earth scientists' best hope for pushing this particular scientific envelope.

For the last great San Andreas fault earthquake, however, we have frustratingly sketchy data. Scientists know of the two M6.0 foreshocks only from a small collection of anecdotal accounts. These accounts suggest, but with a fair amount of uncertainty, that at least one of the foreshocks was centered near Parkfield. We cannot know for certain where these events occurred beyond that they were in central California. Parkfield represents only a best guess based on the fact that the 1857 rupture initiated there.

Although widely felt, the effects of the 1857 Fort Tejon earthquake were modest by virtue of the very sparse population density of the state at that time. We can attribute with certainty only a single fatality to the earthquake: a woman at Reed's Ranch near Fort Tejon who died when her adobe house collapsed. An additional less certain account states that an elderly man fell dead in a plaza in the Los Angeles area.

The temblor had remarkable reach. Its shaking upset bodies of water as far flung as the Kern River, Tulare Lake, and the Los Angeles River. The quake significantly damaged the mission in Ventura, and damage at Fort Tejon itself was severe.

The temblor generated a surface rupture at least 225 miles and possibly as much as 250 miles (360 to 400 kilometers) long, with an average offset now estimated at 5 yards (4.5 meters) and a maximum motion of about 10 yards (9 meters).

Although the 1857 Fort Tejon earthquake hit nearly a half century before scientists would begin to identify fault motion as the source of earthquake waves, the sense of a bisected Earth was obvious even to observers with no scientific training. Stephen Barton, then the editor of the *Visalia Iron Age,* described "a fracture at the earth's surface, continuing in one uniform direction for a distance of some two hundred miles. The fracture presented an appearance as if the earth had been bisected, and the parts had slipped upon each other." Barton went on to observe that "sometimes this sliding displacement would give to the points of hills and to gulch channels a disjointed appearance." Predating the development of elastic rebound theory by a half century and modern fault geomorphology by even longer, Barton's observations reveal impressive observational acuity and acumen.

At this point, having made the trek (at least on paper) from Cajon Pass to Parkfield, let's stop and look back over the expanse of ground we've covered along the way—from Cajon Pass to Fort Tejon, on through Wallace Creek, up Bitterwater Road, through Cholame, and on to Parkfield—at least 225 miles (360 kilometers), a long way to drive. The 1857 rupture, however, tore along this entire ribbon of fault in perhaps three minutes. It shifted real estate over perhaps a third of the state and generated earthquake waves—which make up only a small fraction of the energy associated with earthquakes—felt throughout much of the state. This demonstration of sheer power, nearly beyond human comprehension, reminds us of why earthquakes are not only terrifying but also fascinating. There is nothing like the unbridled forces of nature to put human frailty and foible into perspective.

It all began at Parkfield in 1857. For all its seismological infamy, Parkfield is an otherwise modest and pleasant hamlet, population twenty-seven. Our first clue that the town is something out of the ordinary comes shortly after we arrive and pass a complex of government buildings proudly proclaiming the town's heritage in the form of multiple, conspicuous "USGS" signs.

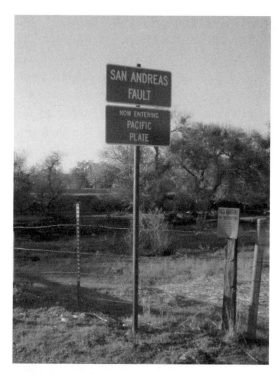

At the bridge leading out of Parkfield, a small sign welcomes drivers to the Pacific plate. (In the other direction, of course, the sign welcomes drivers to the North American plate.)

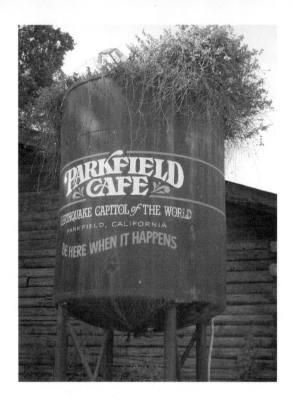

At the Parkfield Café, visitors are invited to "Be here when it happens!" The café menu, like the service, is a delight. (35 54.02N 120 25.97W)

To some extent Parkfield has been a company town since the Parkfield Prediction Experiment began in the 1980s. The terrain is littered with monitoring instruments of every imaginable sort—not only seismometers but also GPS stations, creep meters, gas meters, and more. Although designed to be inconspicuous, telltale signs of monitoring instrumentation abound throughout the town.

Much of the fault trace through the heart of Parkfield is on private property, inaccessible without special permission. A most worthwhile stop, however, is the Parkfield Café, whose menu is sure to warm the heart of any self-respecting seismophile. The neighboring Parkfield Inn invites guests to "Sleep here when it happens!"

Heading north out of Parkfield, we soon reach a low, small ridge on the west side of the road. Here we can find evidence of recent faulting along the lower flank of the ridge.

We leave Parkfield to the north but only by climbing over Parkfield Grade, a winding and narrow dirt road that climbs (and I do mean climbs) over Mustang Peak to meet California 198 some 14 miles later. It is a tortuous 14 miles, not for the faint of heart. However, climbing the grade and finding a suitably safe place to pull over affords a lovely view back toward Parkfield and the valley the San Andreas fault carved. The vista reminds us yet again that the scale of major faults makes them difficult to appreciate at ground level.

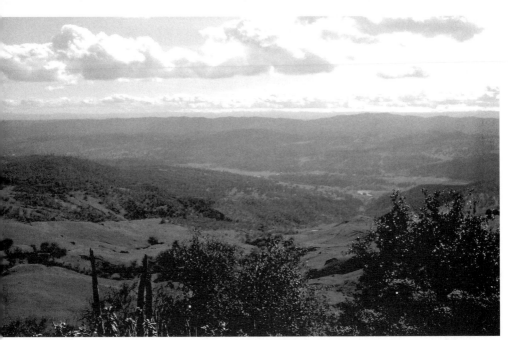

From Parkfield Grade Road, we can look back at the valley, running horizontally across the photograph, along which the San Andreas fault runs.

Dropping down the hill, we arrive at California 198, and not a moment too soon. After traveling 9.8 miles north on this highway, we arrive in the farming community of Coalinga, site of the M6.5 Coalinga earthquake in 1983. The Coalinga earthquake took scientists by surprise to some extent, as it struck not on the San Andreas fault but rather on a blind thrust fault east of the San Andreas. This modest temblor called scientists' attention to the Coalinga-Kettleman Hills, which run just east of the San Andreas, and to the system of buried faults that is accommodating the squeezing associated with the fault. The earthquake was one of those events that, in retrospect, should have been far less of a surprise because fundamental and well-known tenets of earthquake geology tell us that earthquakes on blind thrust faults created the local hills.

No road follows the San Andreas north of Parkfield. We can continue on California 198 to I-5 north, then California 152 west, then California 156 west, which leads to the small town of Hollister. By this point we have passed where the Calaveras fault branches away from the San Andreas and arrived at a location discussed at length in chapter 4: Hollister and the creeping Calaveras fault. Alternatively, we can reach Hollister by taking California 198 west to California 25 north, which follows a course parallel to, but displaced a few miles to the east of, the San Andreas fault. From California 25, we can visit the Pinnacles, volcanic rocks that have migrated some 190 miles (300 kilometers) north from their point

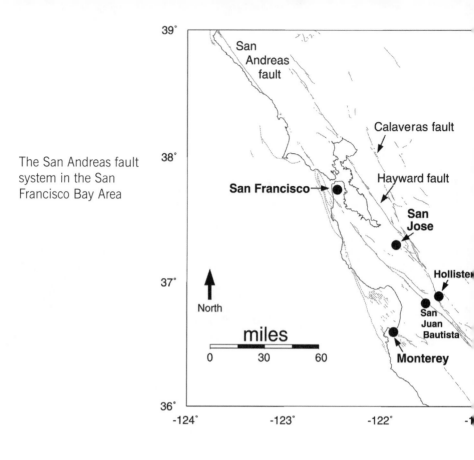

The San Andreas fault system in the San Francisco Bay Area

of origin. Over millions of years, continued motion on the San Andreas fault has separated the Pinnacles from the Neenach Volcanics, a few miles east of Tejon Pass.

Since we have already explored Hollister in chapter 4, this part of our tour will continue a few miles west on California 156 to the lovely community of San Juan Bautista, the southern terminus of the 1906 earthquake. San Juan Bautista also marks the northern terminus of the creeping section of the San Andreas fault, and so fits well in this chapter. But now that our fault-finding tour has reached the end of the creeping section, it is perhaps time to consider some of the interesting scientific issues associated with this part of the fault.

Although the fault experiences some creep between Cholame and Parkfield, the main creeping segment runs from Parkfield north to San Juan Bautista, a distance of more than 60 miles (100 kilometers). Whereas the Cholame-Parkfield segment does rupture in large earthquakes, researchers think the creeping section proper moves only through the more steady process of creep. The creeping part of the fault generates a steady spattering of small earthquakes that illuminate the fault nicely on a seismicity map.

For many years, the locations of earthquakes on the creeping segment lined up in the right direction, but several miles away from the known trace of the

San Andreas fault. This seismological non sequitur proved surprisingly vexing to solve, although many scientists correctly guessed the answer years before it was finally proven.

When seismologists locate earthquakes, their primary data consist of measurements of time: the arrival times of P and S waves at different stations. To determine locations (distance measurements) from time measurements, they must know the speed at which waves travel in the earth. Scientists have gleaned such information in many seismically active places, in greater and lesser detail. In general, seismic velocity increases with depth in the crust because increasing pressure creates more dense, coherent rock. Seismic velocity also varies laterally throughout the crust, in some places with substantial small-scale variability and in other places systematically.

One particularly systematic lateral variation exists across the San Andreas fault in central California. There, millions of years of continued lateral motion have juxtaposed very different rock types—rocks with markedly different seismic velocities. However, most standard methods to locate earthquakes incorporate only a "layer-cake" velocity structure, one that includes variations regarding depth but no variations laterally through the crust. The errant San Andreas fault earthquakes, then, were a consequence of an overly simplistic approach to analysis—of not locating the earthquakes with a velocity model that included the contrast across the fault. When located using more sophisticated methods and velocity models, the earthquake locations scooted over to the fault, where they belonged.

This anecdote illustrates an often overlooked point—that earthquake location is not quite as simple, or as precise, as we might imagine such a calculation to be. Research continues apace on clever methods to improve earthquake location, and to peer into the crust with ever-increasing resolution.

One of the methods developed to improve our ability to locate earthquakes uses arrival-time data from earthquakes that occur very close to one another. Scientists can identify such earthquakes fairly easily by the marked similarity of their seismograms at any given station. Because waves from nearby earthquakes recorded at any one station have nearly identical travel paths through the crust, seismologists can use any small differences in their arrival times to map out the earthquakes' relative locations. Georges Poupinet, from the University of Grenoble in France, and his colleagues first pioneered this approach in 1984. Such an approach can still yield grossly errant locations, but relative locations can be precise within 5 to 10 yards. If that doesn't sound impressive, recall that earthquakes happen deep in the crust, typically 3 miles (5,000 meters) or more below the earth's surface.

But why would anyone want to locate small earthquakes so precisely? Although not consequential events in and of themselves, small earthquakes illuminate

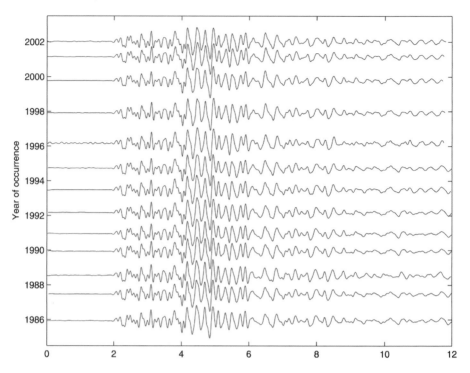

Seismograms from the same station show successive so-called repeating earthquakes. The striking similarity of the records indicates that the earthquake sources are nearly identical. —FELIX WALDHAUSER

fault structure in detail and also provide us with critical information about the processes that trigger earthquake rupture.

Furthermore, some of the most intriguing results from high-resolution studies of earthquake locations have come from the creeping section of the San Andreas fault. For several decades, seismologists have realized that some clusters of earthquakes on the creeping section appear to be carbon copies of each other, producing seismograms at individual stations similar to almost every last wiggle.

Although earthquakes generate very similar seismograms at a given station if the events are merely close to one another, analysis by Felix Waldhauser, Bill Ellsworth, and others suggests that true repeating earthquakes occur on the creeping section of the San Andreas. The favored interpretation is that these earthquakes repeatedly rupture the same very small patches that get stuck as the rest of the fault creeps around them. These sticking points, known as asperities, move only in repeated, small earthquakes. The earthquakes remain small because the asperities are small and because, away from the isolated sticking points, the fault cannot store up strain energy.

Repeating earthquakes on the San Andreas fault are similar to one another and also, in some cases, quite regular in time. These observations suggest that the most simple equations for strain accumulation and release describe their behavior. This realization has led some seismologists to conclude that perhaps large earthquakes behave the same way—that little repeating earthquakes represent analogs for big repeating earthquakes.

However, while earth scientists have solid data showing that some earthquakes on the creeping section of the San Andreas are fairly regular in time, the best geologic data for big earthquakes suggests their behavior is more mercurial. Although the data are sketchy, results from the San Andreas fault suggest that if a given fault segment experiences earthquakes every two hundred years on average, individual pairs of large earthquakes can be as close as fifty years

Felix Waldhauser:
Finding Fault beneath the Surface

Although the locations of small earthquakes can illuminate the geometry and locations of fault zones at depth, standard earthquake location methods typically yield results with far too much uncertainty to study fault structure in fine detail. Through the 1990s and beyond, a number of seismologists, including Felix Waldhauser, have developed sophisticated methods to pinpoint locations of small earthquakes. This is no small feat given that small earthquakes typically occur 3 to 10 miles (5 to 15 kilometers) deep in the crust. Also, the waves from small earthquakes are scattered in complex ways in the earth's crust. By pinpointing the locations of small earthquakes, and sometimes clusters of small earthquakes, earth scientists have been able to not only find faults but also to learn valuable new lessons about how faults and earthquakes behave.

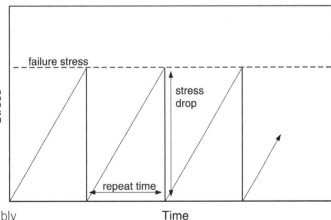

he so-called time-predictable model of arthquakes. In this model, ress builds up at a steady te and is released during arthquakes once stress aches a certain failure vel. Earthquakes are, erefore, regular and redictable in time. This odel appears to describe peating earthquakes, but it oes not hold in general—possibly ecause of the complexity introduced y faults whose cycles affect one another.

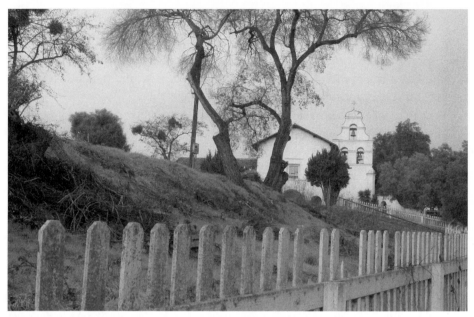

The San Andreas fault creates a low ridge through San Juan Bautista on which the San Juan Bautista Mission stands. The mission experienced some damage but survived the 1906 earthquake, which produced about 6 feet (2 meters) of slip here. (36 50.75N 121 32.09W)

and as far apart as four hundred years—not exactly predictable in a timescale meaningful to humans.

But why would large earthquakes behave so differently than their smaller brethren? Many lines of evidence suggest that the physics of large earthquakes is not fundamentally different than that of small earthquakes. Although scientists don't yet know with certainty, the answer may lie in the degree to which earthquakes "communicate" with one another. An isolated asperity on a creeping fault will be virtually unaffected by small earthquakes elsewhere on the fault because its behavior is wholly governed by the process of creep in its immediate vicinity. On the other hand, researchers know that adjacent locked segments of fault are influenced enormously by large earthquakes on adjacent fault segments and sometimes by earthquakes on nearby faults as well.

New evidence suggests that earthquakes are like a huge three-dimensional game of dominoes in which each large earthquake influences neighboring faults in ways that either nudge them closer or farther away from failure. Earthquakes on large, interconnected faults, then, may not have a chance to establish the regularity of the time-predictable model because they occur on faults whose strain accumulation is too frequently knocked out of kilter by neighboring faults. In the mathematical parlance, such a system is said to be chaotic, the hallmark of a chaotic system being unpredictability.

Still, even if creeping faults cannot provide direct information about the occurrence of earthquakes on large, locked faults, they continue to be natural laboratories for studying earthquakes and faults—including the question of whether creep events precede large earthquakes. Scientists from the U.S. Geological Survey and other institutions have therefore monitored and studied the creeping section of the San Andreas for many years. We may not realize the full fruits of these painstaking efforts until the next great earthquake ruptures the San Andreas fault either north or south of the creeping section, but earth sciences were never a game for the impatient. One of the primary challenges of earthquake science is to be prepared: to establish baselines and deploy instruments so that we can appreciate the lessons that future large earthquakes can teach us.

An additional challenge is to predict the effects from future large earthquakes so that we can design buildings and infrastructures to withstand earthquake shaking. For this, obviously, it won't do to sit back and wait for the next Big One to happen. But to understand earthquake rupture processes, we must collect high-quality data. On both the creeping and locked sections of the San Andreas, scientists have done their best to stay prepared.

Before leaving the creeping segment entirely, one last stop remains on our tour. Creep on the San Andreas peters out just north of San Juan Bautista. To find this part of the fault from the north, U.S. 101 provides a convenient passageway from the Bay Area. Rich with history and charm, San Juan Bautista was along the original route of El Camino Real and is home to the San Juan Bautista Mission. The mission sits atop a low, linear ridge that affords the structure a suitable vantage point overlooking a valley to the east. Unfortunately, the ridge owes its existence to the San Andreas fault—in particular, to the slowing of creep along the fault here.

The San Andreas fault crosses California 156 a few hundred yards east of the intersection with Alameda, the main road into San Juan Bautista. But finding the fault is easier if we proceed along Alameda and turn right on Washington Street to the mission. Approaching the mission, it is easy to understand why Friar Lasuen was drawn to build at this particular site. On a quiet road still lined with adobe structures dating back to the mid-1800s—and with perambulating chickens clucking melodiously around the streets—San Juan Bautista evokes thoughts of an earlier, gentler time. Here again, however, the tranquility is sometimes an illusion. Strolling through the mission to the eastern edge of the grounds, we arrive at the edge of the ridge, perhaps 25 to 30 feet (8 to 10 meters) high here. The main trace of the San Andreas fault runs along the base of this hill and is responsible for its topography. In recent times, the ridge has been used as an outdoor amphitheater, its slope providing stadium seating from which to view performances on the level ground below.

San Juan Bautista marks the southern terminus of the 1906 rupture, which caused about 6.5 feet (2 meters) of slip here. Surprisingly, the earthquake did not destroy the mission. While well built, it is of the traditional adobe/masonry construction known to be vulnerable to shaking. The earthquake did damage it, though, and we can still see evidence of that damage in the structure's masonry walls. However, the modest extent of the damage suggests that the ground motions were relatively modest here.

Recall, however, the fickle nature of earthquake ground motions discussed in chapter 4. That a location was spared (relatively speaking) in one major temblor provides no guarantee that the next Big One—with its own direction of rupture and pattern of slip—will be equally benign. And when the next Big One does rupture the San Andreas fault through San Juan Bautista, far more real estate will be in proximity to the earthquake than was there in 1906.

Heading north on Third Avenue away from the mission, the ridge and the fault remain to the east. Looking east, we find that some of the town's most modern housing was built atop the same rise whose prominence drew the attention of the padres. By the time these units were built, the existence of the fault and the hazard it poses were surely no secret. But the Sirens of California have their call, luring not with music but with the irresistible grandeur of scenic vistas—sweeping views of the ocean or valleys below, views all too often afforded by the offsets along major, active faults.

As we follow San Juan Highway out of San Juan Bautista, the fault is to the east of the road for about 0.6 mile. The fault trace crosses the road near Nyland Ranch, a private ranch where geologist Art Sylvester and his colleagues have carried out detailed creep studies for many years. Nyland Ranch is private property, but we need not venture beyond the road to glimpse the fault's handiwork: an offset fence along the driveway leading toward the ranch. San Juan Highway follows the fault for about another 0.8 mile; then the road bends north away from the fault, which heads off in a more northwesterly direction. San Juan Highway soon leads to U.S. 101 and the Bay Area beyond.

Geographically speaking, central California is loosely defined as everything between the greater Los Angeles region and the greater San Francisco Bay Area. Geologically speaking, it comprises part of the locked southern segment of the San Andreas fault—the part that ruptured in 1857—as well as the entire creeping section from Cholame to San Juan Bautista.

Beginning at Cajon Pass on I-15, the drive through Wrightwood traverses much of the Big Bend, winding its way through and along the base of the San Gabriel Mountains. The northwesterly strike of the fault through this section differs significantly from the direction the plates are trying to move. That geometry gives rise (so to speak) to a substantial component of compression and, over time, equally substantial mountains. Northwest of Tejon Pass, the fault straightens itself out to a direction far more consistent—although not perfectly so—with the plate motion, creating far more gentle hills along the way.

Although we must hopscotch between mainly back roads to follow the San Andreas fault from Cajon Pass to San Juan Bautista, the drive provides ample rewards for the intrepid earthquake tourist—rewards that go well beyond the geological lessons discussed in this chapter. From the pines and alpine setting of Wrightwood, to the thick groves of Joshua trees near Palmdale, to the timeless serenity of the Carrizo Plain and Parkfield, to the rich and charming history of San Juan Bautista, finding faults leads the intrepid earthquake tourist to one postcard-perfect view after another. These scenes are, moreover, at least as remarkable for their diversity—geographical, geological, historical, biological—as for their beauty. (As I drove these roads to do research for this book, I encountered not only the veritable army of ground squirrels but also a sampling of far more elusive wildlife, including wild turkey and an exquisite lone bobcat, who was clearly not used to having his afternoon slumber disturbed.)

To get from Los Angeles to the Bay Area, most people either blast up I-5 as fast as they dare or take the so-called scenic route along the coast. Few people but skiers and campers drive along the base of the mountains between Cajon and Tejon Passes. Even fewer adventurous souls ever find their way to back roads such as California 58, Bitterwater Road, or Cholame Road. Exploring these routes takes time, and, apart from some of the most spectacular evidence of faulting to be found in the United States, their charms are generally quiet and understated.

Yet this neglected corridor is the core of the plate-boundary system that defines California. The sometimes arduous journey from Cajon Pass to San Juan Bautista is a tour through California's past, present, and future—a view directly into its very heart; a view that is far too easily and far too often missed.

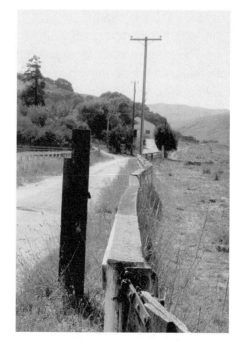

This fence leading up to the (private) Nyland Ranch in San Juan Bautista is offset where it crosses the San Andreas fault. Although this segment of the fault ruptured in the 1906 earthquake, it is now creeping, at least at shallow depths, at about 0.5 inch (1 centimeter) per year. (36 51.31N 121 32.77W)

6 Finding Fault in the Desert

California is known for landmarks of spectacular beauty, cultural and natural alike: the Golden Gate Bridge, Yosemite's Half Dome, the giant sequoias. The elegance of the vast expanses of southern California desert, on the other hand, is easy to miss—especially if viewed through the window of a car traveling 75 miles per hour. From that vantage point, it's hard to notice more than the searing heat, glaring sun, and seemingly godforsaken landscape.

To see more requires closer attention. The desert comes alive on its own terms and on its own time. The wildlife starts to stir as the sun sets: gangly, loping jackrabbits; gracefully scurrying quail; ambling coyote hunting prey. The creatures of the desert are elusive. To find them you must seek out remote trails at quiet times and keep your eyes and ears open.

The most spectacular desert flora, on the other hand, are not hard to find—if you know when and where to look. Many desert areas in California bloom in spring, after winter rains percolate through the sand to summon forth color where it seems unimaginable for color to exist. The wildflowers do not bloom like clockwork, as both their timing and enthusiasm depend on the timing and enthusiasm of the previous winter's rains. In a good year, flowers bloom in some regions with enough ebullience to blanket the ground with golden poppies, bright yellow goldenroot, and lavender Inyo bush lupine. Along sheltered canyons, the more common varieties blend with rainbows of uncommon hues provided by the blossoms on such plants as Indian paintbrush and prickly pear cactus.

The desert's faults, like its wildlife and its beauty, tend toward understatement. However, the geology of the vast Mojave Desert, which stretches from the leeward side of the Transverse Ranges to beyond the Nevada border, is scarcely subtle. East of the Sierra Nevada, lesser ranges stretch northward, defining the Panamint Valley and then Death Valley. A sprinkling of volcanic features, such as Amboy

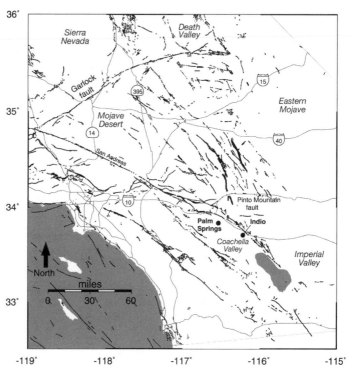

The desert regions of southern California, including the major mapped faults. Dark lines indicate ruptures of the 1992 Landers and 1999 Hector Mine earthquakes. A complex system of parallel faults runs through the Mojave Desert.

and Pisgah Craters, also dot the landscape. Along California 14, Red Rock Canyon rises from the desert floor, an oasis of color with its richly hued and artfully eroded sedimentary layers.

But where are the active faults? During the decades preceding 1992, efforts to find and investigate faults in southern California generally focused on either the San Andreas fault or the faults within the greater Los Angeles Basin. Geologists have mapped faults throughout the Mojave Desert, many of which appeared to be relatively minor. Earthquakes have shaken the Mojave Desert as well, including the M5.2 Homestead Valley earthquake of 1979 and the M5.2 Galway Lake earthquake of 1975. But for the most part, these temblors were small potatoes with modest consequences by virtue of their remote locations. Larger earthquakes in the region, including the M6.0 Desert Hot Springs earthquake of 1948 and the M5.6 North Palm Springs earthquake of 1986, struck on the San Andreas system.

In the late 1980s, geophysicist Amos Nur and his colleagues drew a map of recent earthquake locations throughout the Mojave and suggested that the events represented more than a random sprinkling of earthquakes in a relatively quiet part of the state. Nur suggested that the earthquakes instead reflected the birth pangs of a nascent plate boundary, one that would eventually bypass the pesky Big Bend region and supplant the northern San Andreas fault as the dominant player in the plate-boundary system.

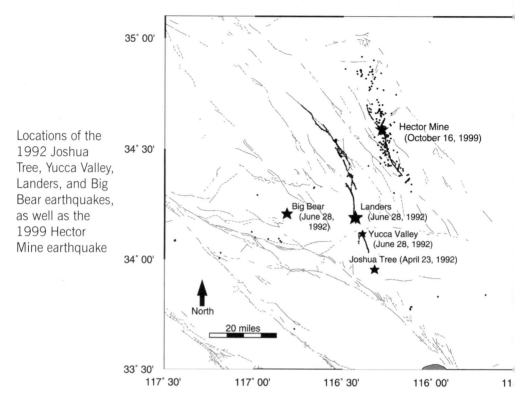

Locations of the 1992 Joshua Tree, Yucca Valley, Landers, and Big Bear earthquakes, as well as the 1999 Hector Mine earthquake

Most earth scientists greeted Nur's suggestion with at best lukewarm enthusiasm. The geologic and paleoseismic records clearly show that motion along the San Andreas has accounted for the lion's share of the plate-boundary motion over the last few million years. The Big Bend clearly does represent a wrench in the works, but, even so, fault systems evolve over timescales measured in millions of years. It will take a long, long time before earthquakes tell us whether Nur's hypothesis is correct—and whether we are, in fact, witnessing the process of evolutionary change.

On the evening of April 23, 1992, the earth added one more moderate earthquake to Nur's list: the M6.1 Joshua Tree earthquake. This temblor occurred within Joshua Tree National Park, a remote area northeast of Palm Springs, and caused minor damage to nearby desert communities. Only harmless, gentle rumblings from the Joshua Tree earthquake reached the greater Los Angeles region some 120 miles (200 kilometers) away. But it sent severe reverberations through the earth-science community, not because of the earthquake's effects but because the epicenter was a scant few miles away from the San Andreas fault. Analysis of seismic data quickly revealed that the earthquake had not ruptured the San Andreas fault, though foreshocks do not necessarily rupture the same fault as main shocks. The Joshua Tree earthquake thus looked like a disturbingly plausible foreshock to a great San Andreas fault earthquake.

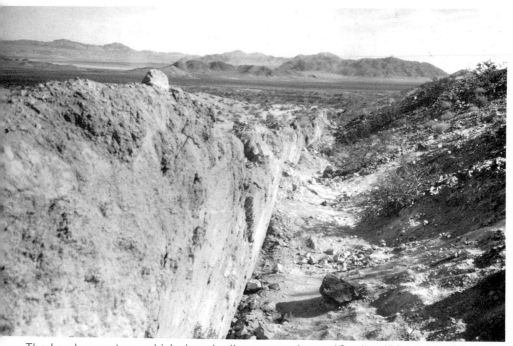

The Landers rupture, which ripped a linear scar almost 43 miles (70 kilometers) long through the desert floor

Over the weeks following April 23, the Joshua Tree region experienced a prodigious sequence of aftershocks—an unusually large number for a M6.1 main shock. Some theoretical and observational lines of evidence suggest that especially energetic sequences of aftershocks occur when significant stored stress remains in the vicinity of a main shock—stress that might then drive a subsequent large earthquake. Given the proximity of the Joshua Tree earthquake to a segment of the San Andreas fault that some researchers have called "ten months pregnant," the energetic aftershock sequence provided little comfort to earth scientists who wondered if a second shoe might still drop.

Near sunrise on the morning of June 28, the second shoe did drop—but not on the San Andreas fault and not on the Pinto Mountain fault, a major east-west trending fault just north of the Joshua Tree area. Instead, the second shoe blasted northward, in map view seemingly a continuation of the earlier Joshua Tree rupture. Within minutes of the earthquake, seismologists had closely estimated both the magnitude and the epicenter of the event. But an earthquake of this size—M7.3—ruptures a substantial length of fault, and the scientists could infer neither the length nor the orientation of faulting from seismic data as quickly as magnitude or epicentral location. One of the earliest clues to rupture orientation is the distribution of early aftershocks, which generally (but not always) delineate the extent of a rupture. Following the Landers earthquake on the morning

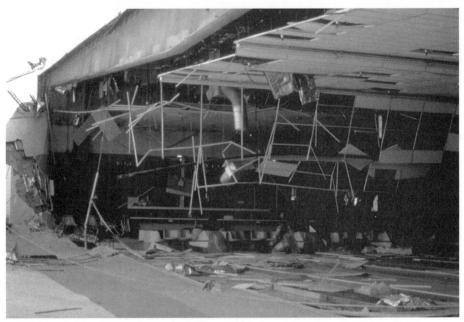

The Landers earthquake damaged the Yucca Bowl bowling alley in the town of Yucca Valley. Engineers attributed the failure of the wall to inadequate connections between the wall and roof. Overall damage from the earthquake was light due to the temblor's remote location, but some buildings in the area experienced significant damage. —LINDA BREWER PHOTO, U.S. GEOLOGICAL SURVEY

of June 28, 1992, aftershocks provided the first hint that the rupture had followed a northerly trend.

But unlike both the Loma Prieta and the Northridge earthquakes, the Landers earthquake announced its presence at the earth's surface spectacularly. Within hours of the earthquake, geologist Kerry Sieh surveyed much of the trace of the fault from a helicopter, documenting its 37- to 43-mile (60- to 70-kilometer) length and dramatic surface features. The earthquake had left a substantial scar through the desert, easily visible even with few roads or other man-made features to document the amount of offset.

The Landers earthquake struck in one of the most sparsely populated areas in California, a happenstance that resulted in remarkably light effects in spite of the temblor's substantial magnitude. The earthquake caused only one fatality, a young boy who had been asleep at the foot of a stone fireplace in a house near the town of Landers. The shaking also took its toll on houses and other buildings in the area, but the impact was far less severe than that of the smaller Northridge earthquake, which struck the San Fernando region two years later.

The remote and arid setting of the Landers earthquake also provided a boon to geologists, who were able to trace the path of the complex rupture along the desert floor. Although the paucity of man-made features complicated efforts to document the precise amount of movement along the length of the fault, teams of geologists eventually mapped the rupture in remarkable detail. The resulting map is almost a textbook of rupture features, with clear evidence of complexities such as branching and the rupture of discontinuous fault segments. The Landers earthquake ruptured several faults that researchers had previously considered discontinuous, and it forever changed earth scientists' views of earthquakes and fault segmentation. Before 1992, academic and consulting geologists thought that the size of an earthquake on a given fault segment was limited by the length of the segment.

Several teams of geologists from academic institutions, the U.S. Geological Survey, and the California Geological Survey (formerly the Division of Mines and Geology) spent weeks mapping the Landers ruptures. Much of the evidence was obliterated, however, in the span of the following decade. Finding faults in the desert is therefore not nearly as gratifying now as it was immediately after the earthquake. This is, moreover, another earthquake tour not well-suited for the faint of heart. Which is to say, the tour is basically in the middle of nowhere—not only far from population centers and points of interest but also not along a route that connects popular destinations. To find faults in the Mojave, a person has to really want to find them. Access to a four-wheel-drive vehicle is also helpful, if not essential.

Fortunately, anyone who doesn't want to venture into the desert can enjoy the tour of the Landers fault vicariously, through words and photographs. To embark

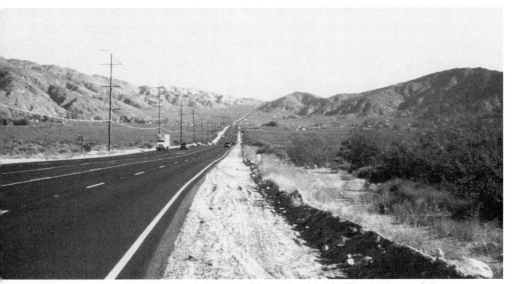

View to the north-northeast along California 62 north of I-10. The highway follows a valley created by the Pinto Mountain fault.

on this tour by car, begin on I-10, east of San Gorgonio Pass and west of Palm Springs. California 62 peels off of I-10 to the north and provides the best local gateway to the Mojave Desert. After crossing the San Andreas fault, a juncture we'll discuss later in this chapter, this stretch of road heads north over the Little San Bernardino Mountains and through the small town of Morongo Valley before veering nearly due east as the road reaches the town of Yucca Valley. The road is a fault tour in itself, as it follows a trail the Pinto Mountain fault cut through the otherwise hilly terrain.

Like the larger Garlock fault to the north, the Pinto Mountain fault trends mainly east-west before it bends toward the south, terminating at or near the San Andreas fault. The Pinto Mountain fault appears to have played an interesting, but not entirely understood, role in the Joshua Tree–Landers earthquake sequence. The fault runs perpendicularly between the fault that ruptured in April and the one on which the Landers rupture began. Looking at a map of both ruptures, we might wonder why they occurred as two separate ruptures instead of a single event. It appears that the Pinto Mountain fault represented enough of a structural complexity to temporarily stall the progression in its tracks. The Joshua Tree rupture clearly amplified the stresses acting on the faults to the north, but those stresses only generated the subsequent rupture after an unknown process of adjustment.

As we drive along California 62, we are therefore driving along the fault that separates Joshua Tree to the south from Landers to the north. It is interesting to consider the long-term interaction of these fault systems because it is not obvious how mutually crosscutting strike-slip faults can continue to exist. The answer may be that they do not coexist in a stable, long-term geometry, but rather that different north-south trending faults are active at different points in geologic time.

In any case, to find the Landers rupture, we head north on California 247 from the town of Yucca Valley. Within a few miles, we arrive in the tiny town of Flamingo Heights. The southernmost Landers rupture ran through California 247 in two locations near Flamingo Heights. Although spectacular immediately after the earthquake, these segments are now hard to find. Even the asphalt is no longer conspicuously fresh from repair. Not too much farther north, however, we turn east on Reche Road and, within 0.3 to 0.4 mile, arrive at a site where we see the fault trace. Just don't expect much. In the aftermath of Landers, the strike-slip rupture in this area was a fresh and obvious tear, but the motion was almost entirely lateral. Recall that geologists rely on offsets in features such as roads and streams to determine the amount of motion in a strike-slip earthquake. In the desert, such features are few and far between. If an earthquake occurs on a strike-slip fault through a patch of desert, it leaves only a thin blade of rupture— in some cases, a so-called mole track—leaving little hint of how much motion has occurred. The ravages of wind and rain quickly obscure such modest features.

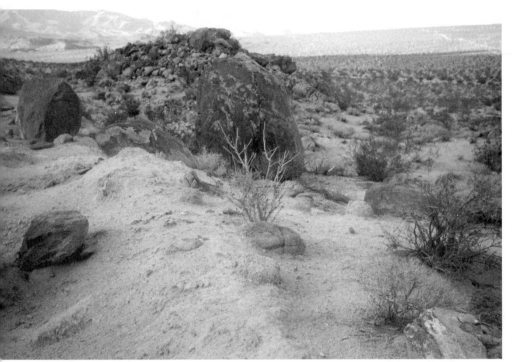

A so-called mole track associated with the Landers rupture. Although the feature is prominent, it is very difficult to tell how much slip occurred at this location.

If we continue driving a short distance east, we arrive at Acoma Road, which runs northward, parallel but slightly east of the rupture.

To find the fault in this part of the desert, it helps to have the assistance of a trained eye—an individual who knows where to look for the subtle but markedly linear remnants of the Landers rupture. At some points off of Acoma Road and other roads in the region, the fault is notable mainly for its accrual of garbage. Tossed out of car windows, the trash blows in the wind before settling in the small linear depression left by the rupture. The process of garbage accumulation mirrors a geologic process in which sediments collect in small depressions left behind by earthquake ruptures.

Nestled among the desert communities in and around Landers, we can find sites that reveal evidence of the Landers rupture, but they are few and far between. One chain-link fence, bent but not broken, remained upright and has been left unrepaired for many years following the earthquake.

Although this region was and still is dotted with modest homes, it was not a site of devastation in the aftermath of the Landers earthquake. The small, structurally simple homes proved to have surprising integrity and did not collapse into rubble even in cases where the rupture ran immediately underneath structures. They did not, of course, escape unscathed. But homeowners repaired damage to

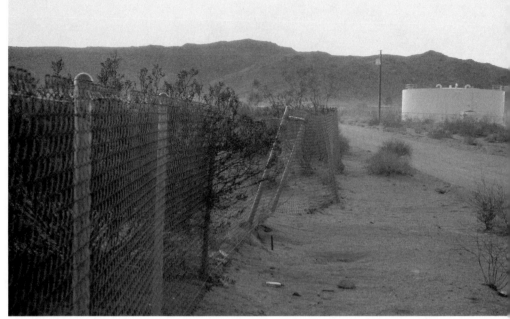

The 1992 Landers earthquake offset this chain link fence on Encantado Road just west of Acoma Road. (34 16.82N 116 26.54W)

dwellings quickly, so homes in and around Landers reveal little hint of the dramatic events of 1992.

To reach the most spectacular fault features associated with the Landers earthquake, we must travel northward to a part of the desert that makes Landers seem like a teeming metropolis. Heading away from Landers on California 247, we follow a route that is largely parallel to, but offset westward from, the Landers rupture. Note that I do not say the "Landers fault," because the earthquake ruptured faults that already had names: Johnson Valley, Emerson, Camp Rock, Kickapoo. These faults extend north-northwest into one of the most desolate expanses of desert in the state—most fortunately, it turned out, because the 1992 quake generated the most extreme ground motions in this region.

The intrepid earthquake tourist can find the fault by following California 247 approximately 35 miles to Bessemer Mine Road, a dirt road that veers nearly due east away from the highway. Primarily used to reach a site for off-road vehicles, Bessemer Mine Road is not exactly a California superhighway and is best navigated in a vehicle with substantial fortitude as well as high clearance. (A four-wheel drive is helpful but not essential.) It is also not a road to be driven in the summer without knowing that the car's and one's own fluid supplies are well stocked. Daytime summer temperatures in this part of the Mojave commonly reach into triple digits, and the desert is not kind to those who venture into it unprepared.

Pressing onward, though, at least on paper, we travel another 7 bumpy miles through Soggy Dry Lake before veering right onto another dirt road. It is called Galway Lake Road, but don't expect street signs. Continuing another short mile, we eventually arrive at our destination: a small hill, essentially a ridge aligned northwest-southeast. Rupture on the Emerson fault cut across one side of this hill, creating the most impressive fault feature associated with the earthquake. At some locations on the Emerson fault, the rupture generated approximately 18 feet (6 meters) of slip, with a small additional component of vertical motion. (Recall that even a predominantly lateral rupture can move vertically as well, especially where faults bend.) At the end of our dirt-road odyssey, we find a segment of the fault that ruptured approximately 15 feet (5 meters) horizontally and up to 6 feet (2 meters) vertically, creating a conspicuous tear that wound its way like a ribbon across the desert landscape.

Immediately after the Landers earthquake, the Emerson fault scarp was a raw and stark stair step, the sharp angles of which contrasted enormously with the desert's windswept features. Within the span of a decade, wind and rain have considerably softened the scarp's blunt edges, but the feature remains dramatic nonetheless.

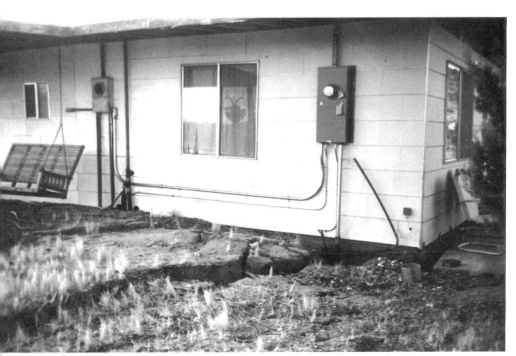

The Landers earthquake significantly jostled but did not destroy this small house, even though the house was built directly atop the fault trace. This may indicate a surprising degree of structural integrity of small, well-built, single-family homes.

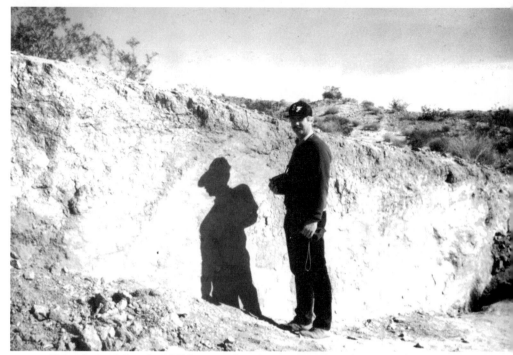

This photo, taken in 1992 soon after the earthquake, shows the fresh scarp caused by the Landers rupture.

Detailed analysis of the evolution of fault scarps suggests that a simple mathematical function of time can describe their degradation from stark stair steps to progressively more smooth ones. After not too many more decades, even the most dramatic features from the Landers quake will likely be quite subtle, little more than a broken linear ridge unlikely to catch the eye of anyone but a trained geologist. Such faults are not conspicuous, but we can find them if we know what we are looking for, as evidenced by the subtle morphology of many Mojave faults that geologists had recognized and mapped prior to the Landers earthquake. But if, as researchers now think, each of these faults produces a major earthquake at most every few thousand years, it will be difficult to identify which of the myriad faults are likely to rupture in the near future.

Nonetheless, geologists have now mapped not only the faults that ruptured in 1992 but also a complex system of mainly parallel faults that spans the length and width of the Mojave Desert (see page 151). The general northwesterly trend of these faults stands in contrast to the Landers rupture, which jumped between faults to create a more northerly path than could have been followed along any one fault. This led to the suggestion that the desert faults have rotated counterclockwise over the last few million years while the orientation of plate-boundary forces drives earthquakes in a direction different than that of the faults. Whether

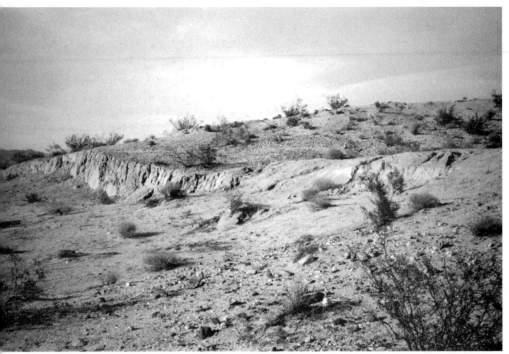
The scarp from the Landers rupture at the same location but nearly ten years later

this process will culminate in newer, straighter faults—and a newer, straighter plate boundary—remains unclear. For the foreseeable future, this part of the plate boundary will almost certainly continue to reflect a complex interplay between past and present forces.

Landers: The Rest of the Story

Although the Landers rupture petered out some twenty to twenty-five seconds after it began, the Landers saga was far from over. Substantial aftershocks, including one that left a 7-mile (11-kilometer) tail of surface rupture south of Landers, began before the main shock's rupture had stopped. Aftershocks throughout the region initially popped off too frequently for the modern Southern California Seismic Network to properly count them.

Among the early aftershocks was a spattering well removed from the Landers rupture, in the San Bernardino Mountains near the resort town of Big Bear. In the chaotic first few hours after Landers, these "stray" aftershocks did not receive much attention from seismologists. In the midst of a fast and furious aftershock sequence, automatic earthquake location algorithms commonly go somewhat awry as P and S waves from different events are confused. Subsequent detailed analysis tends to clean up initially errant locations of aftershocks.

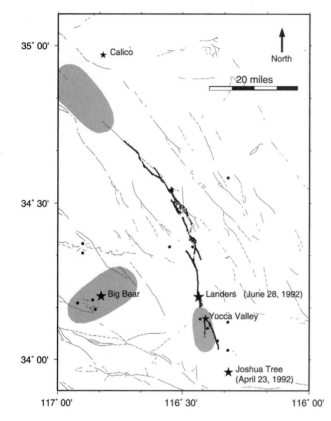

Shaded regions indicate primary lobes of high stress that the 1992 Landers rupture created; small dots mark locations of aftershocks with magnitudes greater than 5.0. The M6.5 Big Bear aftershock, which struck about three hours after the main shock, was centered in one of these lobes, and seismologists infer that stress changes caused by the Landers main shock triggered it. —WORK BY GEOFF KING, ROSS STEIN, AND OTHERS.

However, the Big Bear locations were not artifacts, as the residents of southern California found out minutes after eight o'clock on the tumultuous morning of June 28, 1992. Current theories for stress redistribution after large earthquakes suggest that the Landers rupture created a large lobe of increased stress centered near Big Bear. This stress pushed faults in the area closer to failure, a process whose beginnings were somewhat halting. But at 8:04 A.M. one of the faults failed in earnest. Analysis by then-graduate student Laura Jones suggests that the Big Bear aftershock ruptured two separate, perpendicular fault segments and had a magnitude of 6.5. It was felt throughout the greater Los Angeles and San Bernardino regions almost as strongly as in Landers, and it caused more property damage because there was more property to be damaged.

In spite of the event's substantial size, finding a fault at Big Bear is not—and never was—a fruitful endeavor. Although M6.5 earthquakes commonly do generate a surface break, geologists combed the mountainous Big Bear region and found no evidence of primary surface rupture. They found only a wispy hint of a surface break in this region, displaced several miles from the inferred location of the Big Bear rupture. It is unclear whether this feature reflected minor rupture of a secondary, shallow fault, or perhaps simply large-scale near-surface

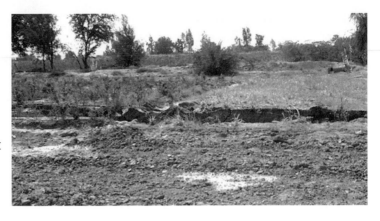

slumping effects. Shaking from large earthquakes is known to cause the ground to slump and deform, simply as a consequence of strong shaking. In some cases, such effects can masquerade as primary surface ruptures.

There is, however, no shortage of faults in the Big Bear area. A system of faults, some parallel to the trend of the Mojave Desert faults and some perpendicular to them, is known to crisscross the San Bernardino Mountains. The best way to find faults in this part of California is to stand back and consider large-scale topography. We can identify the largest faults from large-scale topographic trends: linear valleys and lakes that from ground level appear gentle and serene. Other faults separate distinctly different rock types.

In some ways, the Big Bear aftershock was a surprise, particularly because it struck well away from the Landers rupture. Seismologists now generally recognize aftershocks as events that are not much farther in any direction from a main shock rupture than the rupture is long. However, an earlier, more traditional view held that aftershocks generally strike on the same fault that produces a main shock, not on wholly different fault structures. The Landers sequence provided dramatic illustration of the potential complexity of aftershock sequences, and it heralded the development of significant new theories to explain why aftershocks occur.

But aftershocks large enough to be damaging in their own right were by no means a surprise back in 1992. For example, a large aftershock of the 1952 Kern County earthquake caused damage and fatalities when it struck close to the town of Bakersfield. The Landers earthquake ultimately produced tens of thousands of aftershocks, only one of which generated additional surface rupture—not Big Bear, but an early, approximately M5.6 aftershock that occurred south of the Landers epicenter. According to eyewitness accounts and detailed seismological analysis, this rupture, which did not connect to the southern end of the main shock's rupture, struck about thirty seconds after initiation of the main shock. Although geologists traced the rupture on the Eureka Peak fault for a full 7 miles

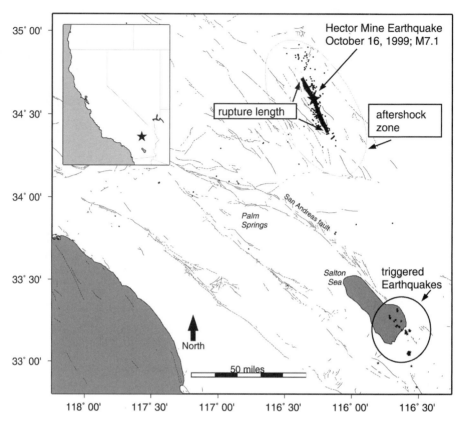

The classic definition of an aftershock zone as well as the remotely triggered earthquakes that followed the 1999 Hector Mine earthquake

(11 kilometers) through and south of the town of Yucca Valley, slip was almost purely horizontal and modest in extent. Erosion quickly all but erased signs of the modest fault features.

An additional chapter of the Landers story was written in the wee hours of the morning on October 16, 1999, when a set of Mojave Desert faults east of Landers ruptured to produce the M7.1 Hector Mine earthquake (see page 152). Aside from being a bit smaller and displaced to the east, the Hector Mine earthquake resembled Landers in many respects. If faults in this part of California rupture every few thousand years or so, the occurrence of twin events within a mere seven years is highly unlikely to have been a coincidence. Yet the physical mechanism by which Landers triggered Hector Mine appears to be complex, related to the slow relaxation of rocks below the brittle crust in response to the Landers main shock. That is, any large earthquake in the brittle crust will cause the material below the brittle layer to shift in response. Sophisticated computer simulations suggest that while the direct stress change that the Landers event caused was insufficient to trigger Hector Mine immediately, the slower process of deep crustal "ooze" did eventually rupture faults in the Hector Mine region.

In any case, like Landers, the Hector Mine earthquake was a boon to geologists interested in investigating detailed surface ruptures of major earthquakes. Seismologists regarded Hector Mine as a guilt-free M7.0 earthquake because it provided a bounty of interesting data to study but caused extremely light damage for an event of its magnitude. (Guilt can be an occupational hazard of earthquake science, as our best data comes from events that typically cause death and destruction.)

Hector Mine was, however, an unmitigated disaster for the earthquake tourist interested in finding faults. Not only did the earthquake hit an even more remote part of California than had Landers, but worse yet the surface rupture was entirely contained within the Twentynine Palms Marine Corps Base. In the aftermath of the earthquake, personnel from the base went to great lengths to help scientists find and investigate faults, even though it meant scheduling fieldwork around highly sensitive and time-constrained military exercises. Researchers, therefore, documented the rupture in great detail and captured it for posterity in innumerous photographs from the ground and air. It is, however, impossible for a casual earthquake tourist—or even an earth scientist without special clearance—to find evidence of this particular earthquake.

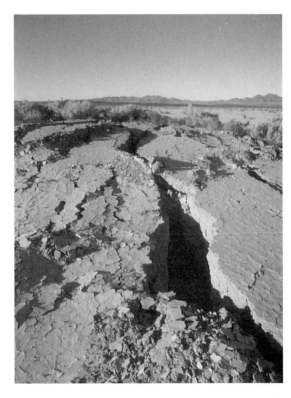

The rupture from the October 16, 1999, M7.1 Hector Mine earthquake
—CHRIS WALLS PHOTO

A Desert in Motion, a Desert in Flux

Relative to a fixed point well east of the boundary between the Pacific and North American plates, the Pacific plate moves northward at a total rate of just under 2 inches (approximately 4.9 centimeters) per year. This motion is distributed across much of the width of California, cutting the state into long geologic ribbons. Researchers think approximately 0.5 inch (1 centimeter) per year of the motion takes place through the Mojave Desert, an area that earth scientists call the Mojave Shear Zone.

Although fault systems and plate boundaries do evolve, this evolution plays out over millions of years. For as long as humans can peer into the future, the overall motion of faults in the Mojave will likely remain well below that of the San Andreas fault. We can, therefore, also expect earthquake rates to be much lower in the Mojave.

But why, the savvy reader might well be asking, have we been "blessed" with such a remarkable bounty of recent earthquakes from faults that do not frequently produce earthquakes? Because, in a word (or rather, three words), we were lucky. Geologic investigations undertaken in the years following 1992 reveal that the complex Mojave Desert fault systems appear to produce earthquakes in clusters separated by a few years or decades, sort of a cascade of dominoes once the first domino happens to topple. In 1992 the Joshua Tree domino toppled on the evening of April 23, and everything else played out from there.

But why did the Joshua Tree earthquake happen in the first place? Good question! If we knew the answer to every good question in seismology it would be a dull science, and (fortunately or unfortunately) we are a long way from that point. Among the biggest remaining unknowns in seismology is the question of why earthquakes rupture when they do—why a certain earthquake strikes at exactly 4:53 A.M. on Monday instead of any other time of any other day. If, as Einstein asserted, God does not play dice with the universe, it follows that He does not play dice with faults either. Which is to say, there must be quantifiable physical mechanisms governing the process of earthquake initiation. We just don't understand them yet.

We can, however, consider the question from another interesting angle. Earth scientists are, as a rule, loath to argue that we happen to live in unusual times. So if we have witnessed a cluster of earthquakes known to be infrequent over the long term, this suggests that there are quite a few faults, or source zones, that produce similarly infrequent large earthquakes. During any given twenty- or fifty-year period, therefore, it is not unusual to see one of them pop off.

Looking back through recent centuries, we find that "uncommon" events have occurred fairly commonly in southern California: Landers in 1992, the M7.3 Kern County earthquake of 1952, the M7.6 Inyo County earthquake of 1872, and a

M7.1 earthquake on December 21, 1812, that may have ruptured the San Cayetano fault near Santa Barbara or perhaps on the San Andreas fault. A bit of grade-school math illustrates the implications: if these "infrequent" M7.0+ earthquakes strike at a rate of approximately one every fifty years, but each such fault produces a M7.0+ earthquake only every 2,000 years on average, this suggests that there are some forty-odd source zones in southern California alone. Modern probabilistic analyses of California's secondary faults, and the hazard that they pose, support this simple "back-of-the-envelope" calculation. The inescapable conclusion, therefore, is that although many of the secondary faults discussed in this book—the Rose Canyon in San Diego, the Sierra Madre and Elysian Park in greater Los Angeles—may individually represent low-probability hazards, but we cannot ignore their combined capacity to produce devastating earthquakes, on par with the 2001 Bhuj earthquake in western India or the 1999 earthquake in western Turkey. Furthermore, while recent "uncommon" earthquakes have struck remote parts of southern California, we must view these events as a dress rehearsal for the inevitable: an uncommon M7.0 to M7.5 earthquake in the heart of one of southern California's urban centers.

Other Secondary Faults in the Desert

Geologic exigencies being what they are, the Landers sequence will dominate any modern discussion of California desert faults. There is nothing quite like a recent M7.0+ earthquake—or several of them—to provide excitement if we are looking to find faults as either a casual tourist or a professional earth scientist. The Landers earthquake sequence claimed a significant fraction of many earthquake scientists' time through the 1990s and beyond because Landers and Hector Mine are among the best-recorded large earthquakes to have ever struck the planet. (The 1999 Chi-Chi earthquake in Taiwan, however, far eclipsed both of them and, by virtue of a major commitment on the part of the Taiwanese government to invest in earthquake monitoring, produced vastly more strong motion recordings than scientists had obtained for any previous earthquake.)

Nonetheless, it behooves us to remember that the northwesterly trending Mojave faults are scarcely the only threats in this part of California. The mainly east-west–trending Garlock and Pinto Mountain faults represent something of an enigma. Geologic evidence suggests both are important faults, with substantial motion in recent geologic times; viewed from the air there is no doubt that the Garlock fault is a major structure. The Garlock fault has experienced a total of approximately 40 miles (64 kilometers) of left-lateral motion over the last few million years. But in recorded history, both the Garlock and Pinto Mountain faults have been quiet to the point of seeming nearly dead. One intriguing study used space-based radar images (InSAR) of the desert to observe directly the amount

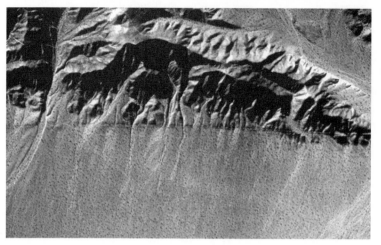

Viewed from the air, the main trace of th Garlock fault stands out as a clear linear feature along the ba of the hills. Geologis Malcolm Clark used photos like this one, taken as part of a U Department of Agriculture aerial photograph series, along with fieldwork to map the full exter of the Garlock fault.

of strain accumulating throughout the Mojave Desert. The InSAR technique, which relies on differences between successive synthetic-aperture radar measures of ground position, cannot be used everywhere but is well-suited for arid desert regions. Gilles Peltzer and his colleagues observed an apparent accumulation of strain along a fault north of the Landers rupture—perhaps the next domino in line—but virtually no strain accumulation on the Garlock fault. The full implications of this study remain enigmatic, as the available data (both GPS and InSAR) only weakly il- luminate the sense of motion expected on the Garlock fault. The data suggest, however, that perhaps strain accrues unevenly on major faults through time, that faults both "turn on" and "turn off" for reasons that remain unclear.

Paleoseismic trenching reveals that the Garlock fault has produced large earth- quakes repeatedly in the recent geologic past, including an earthquake that was probably at least as large as M7.0 less than 500 years ago. To borrow terminology from volcano science, it thus appears that the Garlock fault is temporarily dormant, but by no means dead. Chapter 7 discusses fault-finding opportunities along the Garlock fault because we can easily reach the fault en route to the Owens Valley.

If evidence suggests that neither the Garlock fault nor the Pinto Mountain fault represents a real and present danger, a fault just north of the Garlock fault produced one of the twentieth century's largest temblors in California: the 1952 Kern County earthquake, whose magnitude is estimated to have been approxi- mately 7.5. The Kern County earthquake did not strike within the Mojave Desert but rather just north of it, on the northeast-trending White Wolf fault, which runs roughly parallel to the Garlock fault between the Garlock and the town of Bakers- field. This earthquake might not belong in this chapter, but it is here for two reasons. The first reason involves artistic license: reserving this earthquake for chapter 6 allowed chapter 5 to follow an unfettered tour of the San Andreas fault.

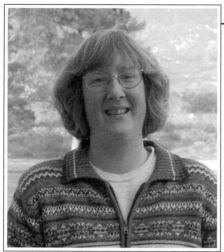

Sally McGill

Sally McGill and the Garlock Fault

Sally McGill recalls a childhood fascination with both maps and landscapes, but no particular affection for rocks. As a graduate student in geology at Caltech, she found herself walking miles of the Garlock fault, spending many long hours looking at rocks. Her fieldwork, coordinated around the schedules of the two military bases through which the fault passes, focused on the smallest identifiable offsets that she could find along the fault. Investigations of large-scale structures and offsets can reveal how much a fault has moved over the long term (typically tens or hundreds of thousands of years), but cannot provide much information about the rate of earthquakes over the last few hundred or thousand years. By identifying small offset features, McGill was able to investigate the most recent earthquakes on the Garlock. She showed that the fault has indeed produced large earthquakes in the not-too-distant past. McGill's results are critical to scientists endeavoring to understand the complex system of faults that run through the Mojave region—they tell us that both the north-south trending Mojave Desert faults (such as those that ruptured in 1992 and 1999) and the east-west trending Garlock fault are active. The Mojave Shear Zone is a complex region and one that researchers do not entirely understand, but McGill's work provides the kind of ground truth without which scientists could not hope to put the puzzle together.

Second, the Kern County earthquake was the Landers of its day, and discussing the earthquake in this chapter provides an opportunity to explore the parallels between those important events. Both ruptured on faults that scientists had previously recognized but not deemed important. Interestingly, both the Landers and Kern County earthquakes were also the first large seismic events to occur in the state after major advances in seismic monitoring. The Landers earthquake followed the installation of the so-called Terrascope stations, seismometers far more advanced than the standard monitoring stations of the Southern California Seismic Network prior to 1990. (Later in the 1990s, the entire network was revamped and upgraded; state-of-the-art seismometers replaced older, less sophisticated instruments throughout southern California.) The Kern County earthquake, meanwhile, was the first large southern California earthquake to strike after researchers

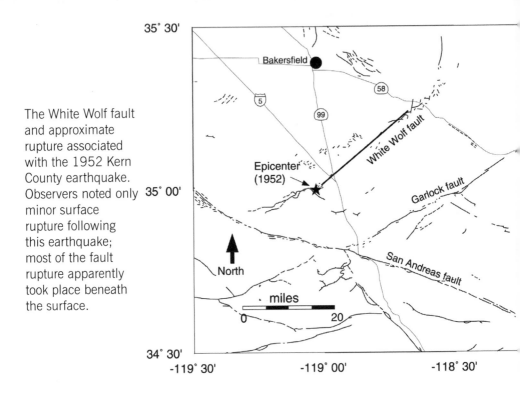

The White Wolf fault and approximate rupture associated with the 1952 Kern County earthquake. Observers noted only minor surface rupture following this earthquake; most of the fault rupture apparently took place beneath the surface.

had installed the first-generation seismic network. The earthquake, therefore, features as prominently in Charles Richter's 1958 classic book, *Elementary Seismology,* as Landers does in this chapter, even though both are relatively rare events. We are left with a philosophical conclusion about earthquake books: if these unlikely earthquakes strike once every fifty years or so, then successive generations of seismologists may write earthquake books that continue the same tradition, perhaps placing undue focus on the saga and the lessons of the most recent uncommon event. We can hope they are at least entertaining stories. For scientists, their lessons have been unquestionably interesting.

Leaving philosophical musings to return to our faults, however, the White Wolf fault had indeed been mapped before 1952, but it had received little attention. In retrospect, Richter identified a series of moderate earthquakes in the general area of the 1952 rupture between 1929 and 1952, but observed that there was, "nothing to distinguish [them] from the peppering of epicenters over much of southern California."

The main shock of the Kern County quake struck at 4:52 A.M. on July 21, 1952—curiously within two minutes of the time of the Landers quake (4:53 A.M.). (Although a number of significant California temblors have struck early in the morning, scientists have thus far been unable to show that this is anything more than a fluke of "small-number statistics.") The small railroad town of Tehachapi felt the temblor's wrath most strongly—twelve people were killed and thirty-five injured from a population of fewer than 2,000. The quake also claimed a handful of lives elsewhere, including a most unfortunate Arvin resident, Ramon Tescado, who was killed by an explosion when he opened the door of his damaged gas-powered refrigerator.

The earthquake also took a toll on buildings and regional infrastructure, leaving an 8-mile section of railroad tracks badly mangled and California 58 torn asunder. However, the surface rupture, which revealed a mixture of left-lateral and reverse faulting, was smaller than expected given the magnitude; apparently the fault moved mainly at depth. Although the toll of the temblor, in terms of both human lives and damage, did not mar the collective California psyche the way the 1933 Long Beach earthquake did, its most sobering lessons come by way of extrapolation. Were a similar quake to strike under the city of Los Angeles, with its three million citizens, and cause a death rate commensurate with that seen in Tehachapi, the death toll would number well into five figures.

The Kern County earthquake certainly did capture the attention of the earth-science community in southern California, as the shaking was felt strongly throughout the region. At the time, seismic monitoring of southern California was the purview of Caltech alone because the U.S. Geological Survey did not receive its mandate to monitor earthquakes until after Alaska's Good Friday earthquake of 1964. When the U.S. Geological Survey did enter the scene, monitoring in southern California became a partnership with Caltech—and later the California Geological Survey—that continues to this day.

In the early days, network seismometers at Caltech recorded on photographic film. On the morning of July 21, 1952, scientists rushed to develop the film and to interpret the signals by hand. In spite of these technical limitations, by 7:00 A.M. Charles Richter and his colleagues had determined that the earthquake had struck 80 to 100 miles northwest of Pasadena. A field team left almost immediately to deploy a portable seismometer southeast of Tehachapi. (Temporary deployments of portable seismometers are common following big earthquakes: they provide key additional data to study aftershocks.) At the time, network seismometers had a limited range of on-scale recording, so researchers used data from these instruments primarily to measure the arrival times of P waves, from which they could determine locations. (Early "strong motion" instruments, run by the U.S. Coast and Geodetic Survey, did record the large earthquakes on-scale.) The sequence of Kern County aftershocks was, therefore, among the first large sequences in California to be mapped in any detail, and produced an energetic spattering of events along the full length of the main shock's rupture, including the M5.8 aftershock on August 22 that caused substantial damage because it hit close to Bakersfield.

Thus was the Kern County earthquake, like Landers, a tremendously important earthquake for scientists of its day. Now that more than half a century has passed, it is interesting to look back and consider the long-term lessons of this event. Kern County represents an important example of a large "unlikely" earthquake in California. In some respects, its importance goes beyond that of Landers in this regard. Throughout the twentieth century, scientists debated whether the secondary fault systems in the Los Angeles region could produce earthquakes with magnitudes well upwards of 7.0—as large as 7.5 or perhaps even larger. Several lines of evidence—including geologic evidence showing that large earthquakes have happened on faults such as the Sierra Madre—seem to have mostly settled the debate by the turn of the millennium. But the very occurrence of the Kern County earthquake—a M7.0+ earthquake on a secondary fault north of the Garlock and San Andreas faults—begs the question of why anyone would have had doubts about similar faults to the south. Were a similar earthquake to occur on a similar secondary fault south of the San Andreas, the consequences and costs would be enormous. The primary impetus for detailed investigations of earthquakes like Landers and Kern County is to understand such earthquakes so that we can better quantify and prepare for similar earthquakes that will someday rattle the heart of California's urban centers.

The Big Fault in the Desert

At its southern terminus not far north of the California-Mexico border, the San Andreas fault peters out gradually. The zone of strike-slip, or transform, motion gives way gradually to a system of smaller transform faults and spreading zones that extend south through the Gulf of California. From its somewhat diffuse point of origin as a transform plate boundary, the San Andreas fault cuts along the eastern side of the Salton Sea before veering west and passing near the Coachella Valley cities of Indio and Palm Springs.

The San Andreas fault exhibits considerable complexity through the Coachella Valley, branching into two segments near Indio: the Banning fault and the Mission Creek fault. The Banning fault is the southernmost strand, and it passes along the southern edge of the Indio Hills, through the valley, and just south of the community of North Palm Springs. In 1986, the Banning fault caused considerable angst when it ruptured in the M5.6 North Palm Springs earthquake, which did not generate surface rupture but did produce a line of cracking along the Banning strand. (Initially, scientists thought these features were a secondary effect of shaking rather than primary surface rupture.) Although the North Palm Springs quake was modest in its own right, earthquakes of approximately M6.0 do not pop off every day on the San Andreas fault, particularly not on strands that some geologists considered overdue for a large earthquake. We do not know what, if any, precursory activity will precede the next great earthquake on the southern

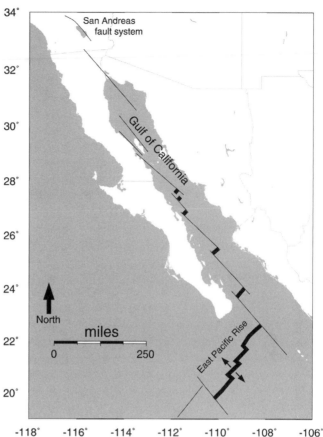

The Gulf of California, a region that experiences a combination of lateral and extensional motion. Straight lines indicate simplified view of faults through Baja California, which include the Cerro Prieto fault and the Laguna Salada fault.

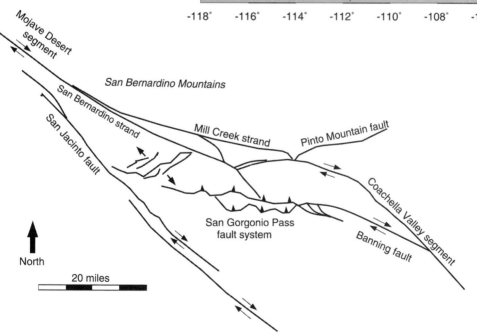

The San Andreas and San Jacinto fault systems in the vicinity of San Gorgonio Pass

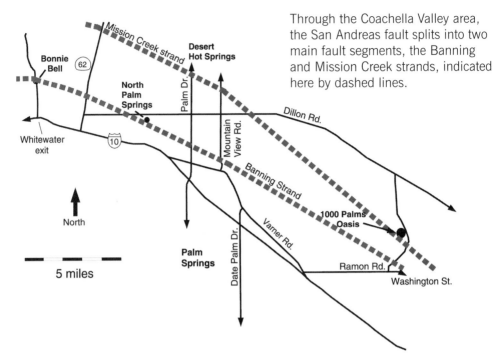

Through the Coachella Valley area, the San Andreas fault splits into two main fault segments, the Banning and Mission Creek strands, indicated here by dashed lines.

San Andreas fault, but a M6.0 foreshock is as plausible a scenario as any. Seismologists think an earthquake of about that magnitude occurred near Parkfield before the great 1857 Fort Tejon earthquake. But the North Palm Springs earthquake proved to be the harbinger of only nerves, as its aftershocks faded away without further ado.

The Banning fault crosses California 62 about 2 miles north of I-10; the fault creates a small ridge that we can trace to the east away from the highway. Farther west, the fault bisects Whitewater Canyon. We take the Whitewater Canyon exit to Whitewater Canyon Road, and after about 1.5 miles arrive at the hamlet of Bonnie Bell, a small, green oasis in the otherwise barren terrain that marks the Banning fault zone. To the immediate east, the walls of the canyon exhibit a broad zone of disruption caused by the fault, which cuts across the canyon at a right angle. To the west, the Banning fault heads off through a cross-cutting canyon that motion along the fault has created.

West of Whitewater Canyon, the strands of the San Andreas fault enter San Gorgonio Pass, known in some earth-science circles as the San Gorgonio Knot because of its geologic complexity. Farther along, both strands of the fault become progressively more difficult to find—even for geologists. The precise location and continuity of the San Andreas fault through this region have been matters of some debate, with some scientists unconvinced that a single through-going fault even exists here. If a single active strand does exist, large-scale landslides might have obscured its surface expression.

A question of tremendous societal importance drives ongoing research into southern California's seismicity: Can a single earthquake rupture the southern San Andreas fault from stem to stern? The segment from the Salton Sea to San Gorgonio Pass has not produced a great earthquake in more than three centuries. The last major earthquake on the southernmost segment of the San Andreas fault happened before the start of the historic record. Geologic evidence points to a rupture around the end of the seventeenth century, when America was but a meager collection of hardscrabble colonies. That segment of the fault could remain quiet for another one hundred years; it could also rupture before this book is published. But eminent geologists identified that segment as overdue for a major temblor before the twentieth century drew to a close. Conventional wisdom, therefore, suggests that it is unlikely to remain quiet for the next five hundred years and is the segment of the San Andreas fault that is most likely to rupture next.

Most of the northern half of the southern San Andreas has ruptured within recorded history, but even in geologic terms, 1857 is not "recent" given the average rate of great earthquakes on the San Andreas fault. This raises the disconcerting possibility that a great earthquake, were it to rupture the Coachella Valley segment, would reach San Gorgonio Pass and encounter a segment with sufficient stored strain to sustain further rupture. Such an event could then continue hundreds of miles farther, rupturing near San Bernardino, Lancaster, and Palmdale, and close enough to the greater Los Angeles region to generate strong shaking there. Geologists have assembled evidence of prehistoric earthquakes at enough

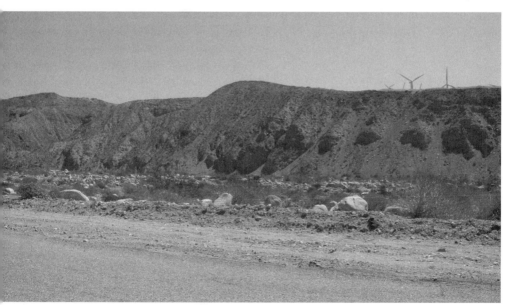

The Banning fault crosses Whitewater Canyon about 2 miles north of I-10, just west of Palm Springs, leaving a pattern of disruption in the east side of the canyon face, toward the left side of the photograph. (35 56.71N 116 38.53W)

locations along the San Andreas to conclude that the southern San Andreas probably does rupture of a piece sometimes, or perhaps in separate events spaced closely in time.

If we contemplate a doomsday scenario for southern California, the maximum earthquake is limited by the maximum available fault area that could rupture in a single event. A repeat of 1857 or 1906 would rupture a ribbon of fault some 250 miles (400 kilometers) long by perhaps 9 miles (15 kilometers) deep. Fundamental physical properties of the crust limit the possible extent of the depth of ruptures on the San Andreas, so earthquakes larger than these events would be possible only were the fault to rupture farther. A stem-to-stern rupture of the entire southern San Andreas fault would be a factor of approximately two larger than the length of the 1857 earthquake. Considering the equations that relate rupture size to magnitude, we find that such a mega-quake could exceed M8.2 to M8.3. That might not sound much different than the Fort Tejon earthquake, which was close to M8.0. But the difference between M7.8 and M8.2 is enormous, especially when we consider the additional population centers that would be close to the strongest ground motions.

Nano Seeber and the Third Dimension

Although Nano Seeber's research includes classic field investigations of faults, he has done much of his fault-finding work on the computer using data from the Southern California Seismic Network. By combining surface geologic observations with "focal mechanism" solutions for tens of thousands of mainly small earthquakes, Seeber and his colleague John Armbruster were able to explore three-dimensional fault structure in vastly more detail than had been possible in earlier studies. Such investigations provide a third dimension to scientists' views of surficial fault structure, information that is critical to unraveling complex tangles of faults in areas like the San Gorgonio Pass.

Nano Seeber at work finding fault in the mountains of southern California
—JAN VERMILYE PHOTO

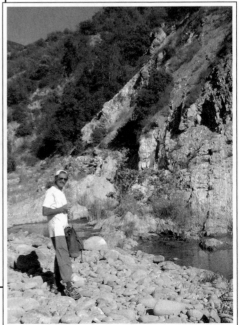

If we were looking to create an even more dramatic doomsday scenario, we could add an additional fiendish wrinkle: a mega-quake on the San Andreas fault could set off a substantial temblor on one of the many secondary faults in southern California, such as the Sierra Madre. As geologist Peter Molnar and his colleagues pointed out in 1996, we can find precedent for such a large, composite rupture if we look at other fault systems around the world. Were a rupture on the San Andreas to rupture a substantial segment of the Sierra Madre fault, the fault area and thus the magnitude, could be larger still. Worse, shaking from the Sierra Madre fault would devastate the greater Los Angeles region—comparable to, if not worse than, Northridge in 1994.

Just for fun, consider another minor variation on this doomsday scene: a M8.2 earthquake tears along the southern San Andreas fault, leaving substantial damage in its immediate wake and moderate damage in greater Los Angeles. Then a M7.5 rupture strikes on the Sierra Madre fault three minutes, or three hours, later—"just" an aftershock, but similar in relative size and location to the main shock as Big Bear was to Landers. Clearly not a pretty picture.

Such scenarios may seem like little more than grist for bad Hollywood scripts, and indeed they do represent very low-probability events. The odds of seeing a doomsday scenario play out in any one lifetime—or century—are low. But earth scientists persist with their efforts to find faults, and to determine which segments might potentially rupture together, because these calculations have important implications for assessing seismic hazard. Ironically, increasing the size of the assumed Big One (i.e., the Biggest Possible One) generally *decreases* hazard estimated in a probabilistic sense. Because truly great earthquakes release so much energy, such earthquakes rarely occur. That is, if the San Andreas system can produce M8.5 mega-quakes, such events might happen only every 5,000 years. Yet these events will release a substantial fraction of the overall energy, leaving less energy to produce M7.5 to M8.0 earthquakes. Meanwhile, modern estimates of hazard generally focus on the earthquakes that we might reasonably expect over any given fifty-year interval—in which case it is typically the more frequent Pretty Big Ones rather than the true Big Ones that control the results. So if we consider this from a standpoint of probabilities, the mega-quakes would be highly unlikely events. If, on the other hand, we assume that the San Andreas generates earthquakes no larger than M8.0, such events would take place more frequently.

The above discussion—the details of which only a mathematician could love—illustrates a few of the issues that occupy earth scientists in modern times, that is, issues that focus on answering questions of great societal consequence. At the same time, questions concerning fault structure and the nature of earthquake rupture also involve enthralling and rigorous science. Faults scare human beings,

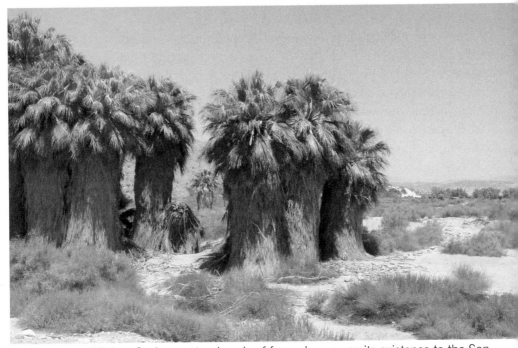

Thousand Palms Oasis, a natural oasis of fan palms, owes its existence to the San Andreas fault, along which water burbles to the surface. (Entrance to preserve: 33 50.26N 116 18.53W)

but they fascinate scientists. Geology is a jigsaw puzzle unlike any other, and one that impels the curious to seek solutions.

Returning, then, to the Palm Springs area, we find ourselves in one of the most congenial places to find faults in California. Not only is the Coachella Valley home to a spectacular fault system, but it also supports little vegetation or human development to obscure the faults' handiwork. However, the San Andreas fault system is not a simple structure through this valley, and following it entails following two faults, not just one.

The strands of the San Andreas fault do alter the Coachella Valley landscape in ways that make them relatively easy to find. In some locations, clays and other minerals within the fault zone form an impermeable barrier, blocking deep ground-water that burbles to the surface along the trace of the fault. Thus, the exercise of finding faults in the desert is often reduced to the exercise of finding trees, such as palms and cottonwoods. Do be warned, however: throughout the region, some trees grow in straight lines because they were planted that way. Not every cluster or line of green indicates a fault.

At a couple of noteworthy locations, we find natural palm oases along the fault, perhaps none more famous than the Thousand Palms Oasis at the base of the northern flank of the Indio Hills, on the Mission Creek fault. To reach this oasis, we take Washington Street from I-10, continuing northward for approximately 3 miles before following the road's westward bend and continuing another few miles to Thousand Palms Road. Thousand Palms Road cuts north through the Indio Hills, leading to the Thousand Palms Oasis in another few miles.

Entering the grove of fan palms at the Thousand Palms Oasis, we quickly step into another world. The magnificent palms provide not only shade but also substantial evaporative cooling as their leaves transpire water. The pools that feed the oasis also bubble invitingly. In the midst of a desert known for sizzling heat, the Thousand Palms Oasis provides a welcome refuge for all manner of life: quail, jackrabbits, lizards, snakes, small rodents, and bats, to name but a few native inhabitants of the oasis.

Human history in the Coachella Valley extends back at least a millennium. In more recent times, the region has been home to the Cahuila tribe, some of whom still reside in and around Palm Springs. In bygone days, the fan palm oasis sustained the Cahuila Indians in innumerable ways, providing water as well as thatch for homes, shoes, and baskets; leaf fiber for rope; small fruits similar in taste to cultivated dates; tea; and even seed pits for use inside of ceremonial rattles. From the days of the earliest human habitation, California's faults clearly played a life-affirming role.

Moving west-northwest from the Indio Hills, the Mission Creek fault follows a course toward the northern edge of the valley and into the town of Desert Hot

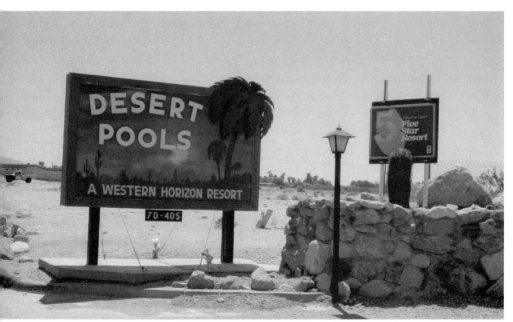

In some locations, natural hot springs burble up along the San Andreas fault in the Coachella Valley, including at this resort near the town of Desert Hot Springs. (33 55.50N 116 25.98W)

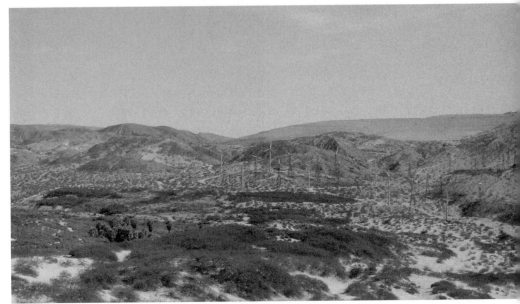

From a hill west of Mountain View Road, the Banning fault trends away to the east-southeast. The clump of palm trees grows along the fault zone, which then follows the gentle valley toward the right edge in the background. (33 53.38N 116 28.54W)

Springs. By now you will not be surprised to learn that both the natural hot springs and the town owe their existences to the fault.

We can reach a good vantage point from which to survey the Coachella Valley faults—both the Mission Creek and Banning strands—by taking the Date Palm Drive exit from the I-10 and continuing 1.3 miles north to Varner Road. Turn left on Varner Road and continue 2.1 miles to Mountain View Road, then turn right and continue about 0.1 mile. Park next to the road. Climbing the modest hill west of the road, we find as much of a bird's-eye view as humans can attain with our feet still on the ground. The Banning fault stretches away to the east, a small palm oasis and other vegetation marking its path before it veers away along a small valley farther west. If we look northward, we see a dramatic, steep, 30- to 40-foot- (10- to 13-meter-) high hill rising from the valley floor: the Mission Creek fault scarp.

For a better view of the Mission Creek fault, we continue on Mountain View Road another 3.3 miles, at which point the scarp looms large indeed. This unusually steep scarp, or pressure ridge, results from a kink in the predominantly right-lateral fault. From here, we return to Dillon Road and drive about 10 miles east to Thousand Palms Road, the northern gateway to the Thousand Palms Oasis.

Returning to I-10, either on Date Palm Drive or from Thousand Palms Oasis on Washington Street, we continue east on the highway to California 111, just

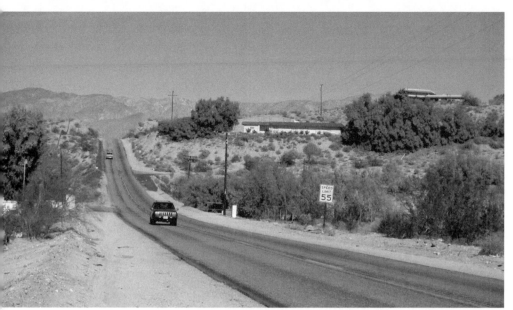

The Mission Creek fault creates a very steep scarp that crosses Mountain View Road north of Dillon Road. (33 56.20N 116 28.53W)

south of Indio. California 111 parallels the (reunited) San Andreas fault, which runs through Coachella and the Mecca Hills to the east. As is the case elsewhere on the San Andreas, linear hills mark the fault where small bends give rise to compressional forces.

After passing through farming communities, California 111 bends toward the San Andreas fault near North Shore, a small community perched at the northeast corner of the Salton Sea. Near North Shore, the fault intersects the highway twice, but its morphology is subtle and difficult to trace. The road meets the San Andreas fault at its lowest point of elevation anywhere along the fault just as we pass the "Welcome to North Shore" sign on the east side of the highway.

At this point, perhaps a few words are in order about the Salton Sea itself. Although something of a cause among environmentalists in recent years, the modern Salton Sea is nothing more than an accident of human ambition and engineering. Over recent geologic time, the region has been home to several ancient lakes, each known as Lake Cahuilla, which filled and dried out several times over. In 1900, however, the Salton Basin (or Salton Trough) contained no water, but its soils were known to be potentially fertile—if only they could be suitably irrigated. Developers and engineers made plans for a canal to bring water to the Salton Trough from the Colorado River near Yuma. Construction of the canal involved a Herculean effort on the part of both men and mule teams to dig a

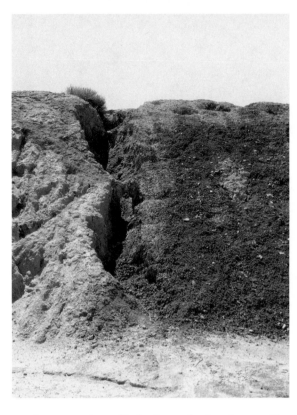

Just east of the Salton Sea and California 111, the San Andreas fault crosses a small gully and railroad switch. The darker (brownish) gouge zone on the right side of the small gully is clearly exposed at this site; a small erosional valley has developed at the eastern edge of the gouge zone. (33 27.43N 115 51.23W)

huge earthen ditch through the desert. The primitive design did not, however, include an emergency shutoff valve. In spring of 1905, heavy winter storms led to heavy spring runoff, and a swollen Colorado River surged over its banks, finding a congenial new course along the freshly dug canal. By July 1905, nearly 90 percent of the Colorado River flowed along the canal system instead of along the river's natural course; three months later, virtually the entire Colorado River was flowing directly into the Imperial Valley. The massive floods and the struggle to control them continued through the spring of 1907, when thousands of tons of rock were dumped to dam the flow. By that time, the Salton Trough had been transformed into the Salton Sea—an expedited reincarnation of Lake Cahuilla.

The Salton Sea's fragility as an ecosystem reflects its unnatural origins. With no source of natural replenishment, the salt content of the water continues to rise. Before its hundredth birthday, the Salton Sea's salinity was two-thirds that of ocean water. There is, however, a tranquil beauty to the sea, its waters varying from turquoise to deep cobalt against a muted, windswept backdrop. The sea has become a haven for migratory waterfowl attracted to the open water and marshlands. Thousands of birds, including Canada geese, pelicans, and grebes, use the Salton Sea as a migratory pit stop or a winter home. The fate of the sea, as well as its role as a haven for waterfowl, does not appear promising. Inescapably, the desert is destined to reclaim the land it lost.

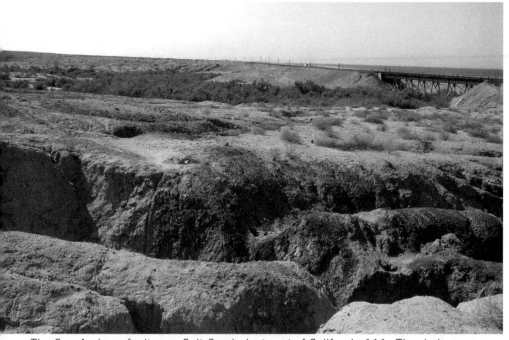

The San Andreas fault near Salt Creek, just east of California 111. The dark gouge zone is again clearly exposed (more so in color than in black and white) where the fault crosses a gully just north of Salt Creek. (33 26.92N 115

Skirting the shore along California 111, the fault passes east of the road. Continuing less than 5 miles south of North Shore, we arrive at a nondescript bridge (marked 56-0281) just west of a culvert that crosses the railroad tracks to the east of the road. The easiest way to distinguish this particular bridge and culvert from all the others is with a GPS receiver (33 27.37N 115 51.56W). Parking off the road and crossing the railroad tracks (carefully!), we find a railroad switch that bends off the north-south line, veering nearly due east. Tracking this switch to its point of termination, we follow a small gully, the walls of which eventually expose an impressive exposure of the fault. In this light-colored terrain, brownish rock indicates a thick gouge zone, the eastern edge of which is clean and straight. Strictly speaking, the entire gouge zone—not just one edge or the other—is the fault.

Strolling about 0.5 mile due south of this site, we arrive at Salt Creek (33 26.89N 115 50.72W), a drainage whose geometry has been shaped by long-term motion on the fault. Some 120 miles (200 meters) east of the road, where the fault crosses a gully, the brown gouge layer is again well exposed.

South of Salt Creek, near the small town of Durmid, a broad hill called Durmid Hill rises from the desert floor to the east of California 111. Pressure from the San Andreas fault is pushing Durmid Hill upward at a rate of approximately 0.16 inch (3 millimeters) per year. Dark ridges atop Durmid Hill are known as Bat Cave

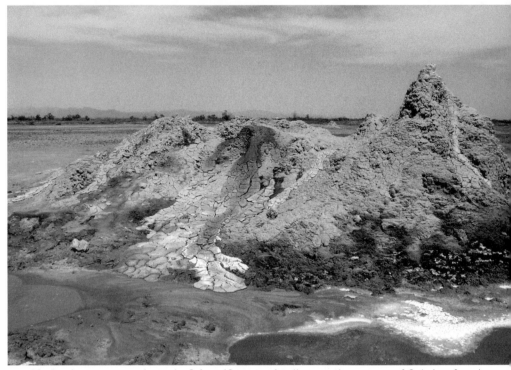

Mud volcano, approximately 6 feet (2 meters) tall, near the corner of Schrimpf and Davis Roads in Niland.

Butte. Just a few thousand years ago, these hills were an island poking its head above the surface of ancient Lake Cahuilla. (The lake apparently dried out slowly, disappearing altogether only about 400 years ago.)

As we approach the small community of Bombay Beach, California 111 bends toward the northeast and crosses the San Andreas, but the fault is hard to find because it creates only subtle surface features in this location. Thus does the San Andreas fault reach an end, not with a bang but with a whimper: at Bombay Beach, where the contour of the Salton Sea bows out toward the east. Beyond here, the fault zone quickly becomes fuzzy. Earthquake locations delineate a band of activity through and beyond the Salton Sea, the so-called Brawley Seismic Zone. This zone appears to be associated with a complicated mix of lateral and extensional tectonics, reflecting the transition from a transform to a spreading plate boundary. Extension to the south of the Salton Sea and beneath its waters has given rise (so to speak) to recent volcanic and geothermal activity. An active geothermal field operates immediately south of the Salton Sea, tapping the earth's surfeit of heat to generate electricity.

We reach the southernmost stop on our grand tour of California by following California 111 through Niland to Davis Road, which leads to the Wister State

Wildlife Refuge (also known as the Imperial Wildlife Area). Following Davis Road south for just under 6 miles to the corner of Davis and Schrimpf Roads, we arrive at the corner of a field in which a remarkable crop is growing: mud volcanoes. (Alternatively, we can reach this site by taking California 111 south, past McDonald Avenue, to Schrimpf, and turning west.)

Mud volcanoes are what their name implies: volcanoes fed not by magma but by reservoirs of deep-seated geothermal fluids that burble up from depth, mixing with sediments along the way to make a gray, soupy mud. Given the inconsequential nature of mud, these features do not grow to more than 6 to 10 feet (1 to 2 meters) tall, and so arguably do not live up to the grandiosity of their names. They are nonetheless enchanting features, each burping mud with a unique rhythm and tone governed by their ever-changing internal geometry and level of activity. Mud volcanoes sometimes sleep, but they wake with gentle and surprising songs.

A few miles west of these mud volcanoes, we can find evidence of volcanism on a far grander scale: Red Island, a volcanic dome that erupted approximately 16,000 years ago. This dome and other evidence of volcanic activity stand in testimony to the extensional processes at work south of the Salton Sea.

Farther south in the Imperial Valley, south of the Salton Sea, faulting continues to be both diffuse and complex. Near the town of El Centro, we rejoin a well-developed segment of strike-slip faulting in the form of the Imperial fault, which is one of those California faults that has called attention to itself in recent times, in this case twice in the twentieth century alone.

On May 19, 1940, the Imperial fault ruptured both north and south of the international border, a 37-mile (60-kilometer) stretch of mainly right-lateral rupture that produced a M7.1 earthquake. This earthquake is especially noteworthy because it was the first major temblor to be recorded by a strong-motion instrument right next to the fault. The resulting strong-motion record provided clear evidence for the complexity of earthquake ruptures.

Researchers deployed additional instruments in the region in the years following 1940. Their efforts were rewarded in spades on October 15, 1979, when the Imperial fault ruptured again. This time the rupture was confined to the approximately 19-mile (30-kilometer) stretch of fault north of the United States–Mexico border, producing a commensurably smaller earthquake of M6.5. Curiously, however, the pattern of slip from the 1979 earthquake was nearly identical to that observed on this part of the fault in 1940. That is, while the two earthquakes ruptured different lengths of the fault and thus had different magnitudes, the northern part of the fault had a very similar rupture pattern in 1940 and 1979. This has led to speculation that a given segment of fault might not always rupture in identical earthquakes, but might instead be associated with a "characteristic slip" that occurs on that segment from event to event. According to this model, a particular fault segment might always experience, say, 10 feet of slip, but sometimes as part of earthquakes that include other fault segments, and sometimes on its own.

If the characteristic slip model seems confusing, imagine two checkers on the back row of a checkerboard advancing forward according to the following rules: the first checker can move directly forward by one square at a time, and the second checker can move directly forward two squares at a time. The checkers can move independently or at the same time, but only by their allotted increments. The checkers can reach the end of the board at the same time if the one-hop checker moves more frequently than the two-hop checker. Thus can adjacent fault segments eventually move by the same total amount, while each moves by a different "characteristic" amount in each earthquake.

Aron Meltzner: Finding Fault in Farm Country

As a graduate student at San Diego State University and Caltech, Aron Meltzner has been finding fault in the Imperial Valley, hoping to uncover evidence of prehistoric earthquakes on the faults that connect the Gulf of California spreading center to the San Andreas fault. Although of tremendous importance, researchers have not previously studied these faults in detail largely because they are so hard to find. Farming activity has not only scraped clean much of the recent sedimentary layers that might have contained evidence of past earthquakes, but they have also outright leveled fault features created as recently as 1979. Meltzner tells of visiting a site known to have had a small vertical offset in 1979 and finding no evidence of the fault trace—only an offset between one agricultural field and the next. By leveling the field through which the fault ruptured, the farmer essentially shifted the fault scarp from its original location to the border between two fields. As if faults weren't difficult enough to find without being moving targets!

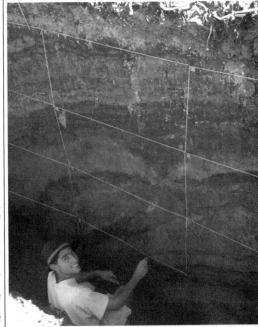

Aron Meltzner smiles up from the bottom of a trench across the San Jacinto fault. By examining the near-surface sediment layers, geologists can infer the amount of motion and the timing of prehistoric earthquakes on a fault.

In any case, the 1979 earthquake provided not only a relative wealth of data for seismologists but also a surface rupture that geologists mapped in detail. The rupture cut through an agricultural region, so scientists could trace it in several places from a systematic disruption of once-linear rows of crops. Within a few scant decades, however, not only erosion but also the abundant and energetic farming activities in the region largely obliterated evidence of the 1979 rupture.

The southern Salton Sea, Imperial Valley, and the northern Gulf of California all experience high rates of seismicity, including small, moderate, and occasionally big events. The hot and thin crust in this region appears to predispose the area to innumerous swarms of small events as well as fairly frequent larger earthquakes. But the thin, hot crust appears unable to store sufficient strain energy to generate great earthquakes. It is possible that earthquakes might originate in or north of the Imperial Valley and propagate to the San Andreas. Additional investigations such as those initiated by Meltzner and Rockwell should reveal whether such events have happened in the past.

The southern terminus of the San Andreas fault has been the cause of some concern—or rather, consternation—over the years. Faults in this region have repeatedly experienced "triggered slip" following large earthquakes in southern California. Triggered slip is movement on faults, typically in the upper few miles, that follows large regional earthquakes. The 1999 Hector Mine earthquake generated not only triggered slip but also a sequence of triggered

Michael Rymer and Triggered Slip

Mike Rymer has spent decades studying faults in the deserts of southern California. Among other fault-mapping endeavors, Rymer has documented and measured a phenomenon known as triggered slip, whereby sections of one fault will move a small amount when earthquakes strike on other faults. Along the southern San Andreas fault, triggered slip has happened repeatedly on certain segments—but not on other segments—following earthquakes such as the 1992 Landers and the 1999 Hector Mine earthquakes. Whereas fault mapping is not generally a time-critical endeavor—in the sense that faults can be mapped as well tomorrow as today—observations of triggered slip must be made in the immediate aftermath of earthquakes so that researchers can be sure of the timing of the slip. With his home base at the U.S. Geological Survey's western regional headquarters in Menlo Park, Rymer has been fortunate (some might say unfortunate) enough to have been "pre-deployed," or already in the field, for a couple of the large earthquakes that struck the southern California desert in the 1990s. The data that Rymer has collected provides insight into the nature of faults: the conditions that nudged them to move (slightly), and the conditions that allow them to remain stubbornly still.

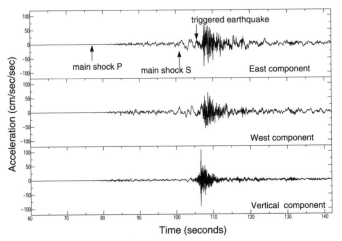

Seismogram recorded near the southern end of the Salton Sea during the M7.1 Hector Mine earthquake of October 16, 1999. The large signal toward the end of the record indicates a separate earthquake that struck close to the station—triggered by the waves from the Hector Mine temblor's main shock.

earthquakes near the Salton Sea, beginning with a M4.6 earthquake that struck immediately on the heels of shaking from the Hector Mine quake's main shock. We don't know what, if any, precursors will precede the next great earthquake on the southern San Andreas fault, but here again the scenario that played out in 1999 was a disturbingly plausible precursor. And, once again, nothing happened. Where the identification of earthquake precursors is concerned, it is clearly not enough to simply find fault. We have to understand them as well.

In 1989, geophysicist Ken Hudnut and his colleagues identified one potential mechanism for triggering earthquakes on the San Andreas fault. Observing that a M6.2 earthquake on a northeast-trending fault in 1987 was followed approximately twelve hours later by the M6.6 rupture of the Superstition Hills fault just southwest of the Salton Sea, Hudnut proposed a mechanism known as cross-fault triggering. The idea behind this mechanism is conceptually straightforward: rupture on one fault can relieve the "clamping" stress on a longer fault oriented in a perpendicular, or "conjugate," direction, thereby triggering a subsequent event.

Hudnut and his colleagues further speculated that the fault that triggered the Superstition Hills earthquake was only one of a system of northeast-trending cross faults in the region, and that a more northerly cross fault could someday rupture and detonate the Big One on the San Andreas.

Scientists have greatly expanded and developed the idea behind cross-fault triggering in the aftermath of the 1992 Landers earthquake. They have made enormous strides in understanding the complex stress changes associated with large earthquakes, and the effects these stress changes have on subsequent earthquakes. Whether these events will be manifest in the precursory sequence, if any, that precedes the next great San Andreas fault earthquake remains to be seen. If, however, a rupture of approximately M6.0 were to occur on a northeast-trending cross fault under the Salton Sea, we would have a documented physical basis for viewing (and worrying about) the event as a possible precursor.

The Superstition Hills fault is one of a series of faults that extends northwest from El Centro: first the Superstition Hills and Superstition Mountain faults, then the Coyote Creek and the San Jacinto faults. The most important of these, the San Jacinto, runs through the Anza-Borrego Desert before continuing on toward San Bernardino. The relatively short Coyote Creek fault, now considered to be part of the San Jacinto system, ruptured to produce the M6.5 Borrego Mountain earthquake of 1968.

Although the San Andreas fault eclipses it in fame, the San Jacinto fault system has been one of the most active faults in California in recorded history. Seismologists have identified one segment of the San Jacinto, near the small town of Anza, as a likely seismic gap—a stretch of fault that has not ruptured significantly for some time and that might be considered overdue.

Around 1980, seismologists installed a specialized array of seismic monitoring instruments in the Anza area, instruments that were, at the time, exceptionally sophisticated. The motivation for this array was twofold: to monitor a region considered likely to produce a moderate (M6.0 or larger) earthquake; and to record earthquakes at sites situated on extremely hard granitic rock. Historically, the

Tom Rockwell and the San Jacinto Fault

Paleoseismologic investigations in southern California have primarily focused on the San Andreas fault. However, the prehistoric earthquake record on the San Jacinto fault, which arguably rivals the southernmost segment of the San Andreas in its rate of slip and earthquake production, is far less well understood. Tom Rockwell has identified a site that may represent "the Pallet Creek of the San Jacinto fault": Hog Lake, in the mountains near Anza, contains sedimentary evidence of at least ten major, surface-rupturing earthquakes on the San Jacinto fault during the past 3,000 years. Although the structure of the fault itself is fairly well known, in this case the neat trick was finding the site from which to study the fault. The Hog Lake site is underwater most of the time. Only after the driest winter in decades did the site dry out enough to allow Rockwell and his colleagues to embark on an investigation. Even then, only vigorous and continuous pumping kept the trench from flooding. The work may have been daunting, but the potential rewards are enormous. Scientists continue to debate the extent to which the plate boundary is distributed between the southernmost San Andreas fault and the San Jacinto fault, with some lines of evidence suggesting that each fault system accommodates about half of the plate motion. Rockwell's results—still a year or two away at the time of this writing—should provide critical new data to help settle the issue.

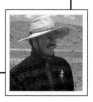

Geologist
Tom Rockwell

dampening, or attenuation, of earthquake waves after they leave the source has greatly hampered attempts to understand the detailed process of earthquake rupture—that is, what really happens on a fault during an earthquake. It's a little like listening to music piped through an equalizer with skewed and unknown settings and trying to reconstruct both the original tune and the settings of the equalizer. But as is so often the case, the earth's lessons included humility. Detailed investigations using Anza data (including this author's Ph.D. thesis) revealed that we could not easily discern earthquake sources with Anza data, as seismic waves were significantly attenuated in even so-called hard rock. Moreover, the Anza gap remained stubbornly unfilled for twenty years and counting after researchers installed the array of monitors.

There is, however, little doubt regarding the hazard the San Jacinto fault poses, and the Anza gap represents only the tip of the iceberg. Whereas near and south of Anza the fault runs through lightly populated mountain and desert regions, toward its northern terminus it runs into the growing megacity of San Bernardino. By virtue of being a relatively young and highly segmented fault, the San Jacinto

Steve Wesnousky and the Maturity of Faults

With a background in both geology and seismology, Steve Wesnousky has explored the nature of faults by investigating the earthquakes that occur on them. The magnitudes of earthquakes in any given region (not a given individual fault) are known to follow a fairly simple pattern: there are roughly ten times the number of M5.0 events as M6.0's, and ten times the number of M4.0's as M5.0's, and so on. Looking at the magnitudes of earthquakes on individual faults, Wesnousky concluded that earthquakes on fairly young, "immature" faults such as the San Jacinto follow this pattern, but earthquakes on older, "mature" faults such as the San Andreas do not. According to Wesnousky's results, mature faults tend to rupture in large earthquakes, without producing smaller earthquakes at

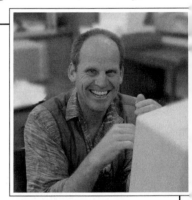

Steve Wesnousky hard at work in his office —Courtesy of Steve Wesnousky

the rate the usual equations predict. For example, a section of the San Andreas might produce an earthquake of approximately M8.0 every two hundred years, but, in that span of time, far fewer than ten quakes of approximately M7.0, one hundred quakes of approximately M6.0, etc. Such an analysis does not find fault per se, but rather provides a characterization of faults that has important implications for hazard assessment.

fault may generate relatively more Pretty Big Ones than the San Andreas. While the odds of a great earthquake on the San Jacinto might be low, the 1994 Northridge earthquake provided a stark illustration of the havoc that a Pretty Big One can wreak if it strikes close to population centers.

The San Jacinto fault emerges from the relatively sparsely populated environs of Riverside County and enters San Bernardino County just east of Reche Canyon. From there, it threads the needle formed by the I-215/I-10 interchange in Colton, just south of the Santa Ana River. A major earthquake on the northern San Jacinto fault would clearly not do good things to this heavily trafficked crossroads, but Cal-Trans engineers have taken pains to retrofit the interchange as well as current technology allows. Retrofitting of interchanges typically involves wrapping the columns in steel jackets and in some cases designing a segmented roadbed that can accommodate movement between adjacent segments. The California Geologic Survey has also instrumented the interchange with an impressive assortment of seismometers that record shaking at not only the ground level but also on the structure itself. These impressive efforts notwithstanding, being located directly atop a major fault is clearly not ideal for a major freeway interchange.

To find faults in this area, we embark on a short driving tour near the interchange. From I-10, we exit onto Waterman Avenue and head south to Commercial

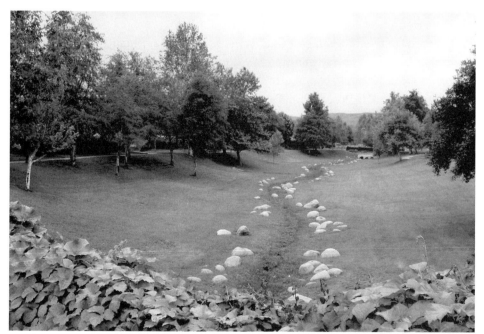

Just south of I-10 in San Bernardino, a lovely greenway marks the San Jacinto fault zone, which is unbuildable under the Alquist-Priolo Act. The fault itself created the little valley; the pretty landscaping is a recent modification. (34 03.48N 118 17.11W)

Road. Approximately 0.2 mile before Commercial Road reaches Hunts Road, we cross the trace of the San Jacinto fault. Here, the fault is not hard to find. Unbuildable by virtue of the Alquist-Priolo Act, this part of the San Jacinto fault zone now serves as a greenway cutting through residential neighborhoods, one of the more charmingly landscaped fault zones in California.

North of the greenway, the fault crosses the Southern Pacific railroad line before reaching the interchange. To follow the fault, take Hunts Road west to E Street, then E Street north to Orange Show Road. Turning left (west) on Orange Show Road, we rejoin the San Jacinto fault 0.4 mile after passing under I-215. Radio towers just south of Orange Show Road are within the fault zone. Farther ahead in San Bernardino, the fault bisects San Bernardino Community College, where engineers have devoted significant attention to reducing the risk to campus buildings. A fault scarp along the San Jacinto fault is visible on the south side of campus, on Grant Avenue about a block east of Mt. Vernon Avenue.

The Elsinore fault parallels the San Jacinto but is displaced to the west. It passes through the valley that is home to the growing communities of Temecula and Lake Elsinore, among many others. Approaching the greater Los Angeles region, the Elsinore fault appears to feed into the Whittier–Elysian Park fault, although the degree of connectivity between the two systems is not entirely clear.

Considering a map of southern California's faults, and thinking about what the plate boundary "ought to" look like, we have to wonder again if the plate-boundary system is in a state of flux. Perhaps as the San Jacinto fault continues to develop (becoming more mature) it will eventually supplant the southern San Andreas as the primary plate-boundary fault. Perhaps someday but—as is the case for the Mojave Desert faults—not today and not any time soon.

Fault systems develop and evolve over geologic time, which is nearly incomprehensible to the human mind. We can only piece together the past and gaze into the future through the murkiest of crystal balls. For the purposes of quantifying earthquake hazard, however, geologic time is irrelevant. We worry about the earthquakes that might happen over the next thirty or fifty years, not those that will strike 3 million years from now. But if we seek to understand the intricate complexities of the plate-boundary system, the evolution of faults provides a most intriguing additional dimension to the already complex, and fascinating, puzzle: the dimension of time.

It may seem contradictory that scientific issues related to the temporal evolution of the California plate-boundary system figure so prominently in this chapter, which focuses on faults in the most seemingly timeless part of the state. But like the terrain itself, there is far more to desert geology than first meets the eye. If we listen and look carefully, its earthquakes and faults stand to tell us much about not only earthquake hazard but also about the enormous, richly complex jigsaw puzzle that is California.

7 Finding Fault in the Owens Valley

The Owens Valley is another of California's underrated corridors, most commonly viewed from a car window while traveling as fast as legally, and logistically, possible. From U.S. 395, it's easy to overlook the subtle charms of the Owens Valley—especially if we are preoccupied with the slow-moving RV in front of us or the ski-laden SUV closing fast in our rearview mirror.

But if you slow down and give it half a chance, the Owens Valley, like other desert regions, comes to life historically, culturally, and geologically. Although sparsely populated in modern times, the region experienced the boom and bust of California's early days as a mining state. A modest gold strike near Bridgeport Valley in 1857 set off the first gold rush on the east side of the Sierra Nevada, though not all that glittered was gold. Less than a decade later, in 1865, the richest silver strike in the state was made at Cerro Gordo in the Inyo Mountains. The region's largest gold strike, meanwhile, was made in the Bodie Hills east of Mono Lake. The town of Bodie—named for prospector William S. Bodey—quickly swelled to 6,000 inhabitants. A scant two decades later, however, Bodie was approaching its current ghost town status.

The mining heyday marked the end of a way of life for the Owens Valley's seminomadic Paiutes, who had inhabited the region for at least 1,000 years. (The Paiutes spoke the language of the Shoshones, and are sometimes known as the Paiute Shoshones.) Following an all-too-typical series of tensions and conflicts, about nine hundred Paiutes surrendered to U.S. Army forces in 1863 and were relocated to a reservation near Fort Tejon.

Some of the most captivating rock sites in the Owens Valley have nothing to do with geology and everything to do with the region's earliest human inhabitants. About 5,000 years ago, forerunners to the Paiutes etched intriguing petroglyphs into boulders at a number of locations throughout the Owens Valley. Unfortunately, it is not as easy to find some of the best sites as it once was because access has been restricted. Their existence, however, serves as a poignant reminder that history documented by settlers of European descent represents the blink of an eye compared with the timescale over which forces have shaped the Owens Valley. Had the history of the Paiutes and their forerunners been better recorded and preserved, we would know far more about not only the first human inhabitants themselves but also about the earthquake history of the region they called home. The meaning and purpose of the only surviving written record—the petroglyphs— remain enigmatic. They have not previously been interpreted to describe earthquakes, but the idea is not far-fetched.

Some Paiute legends have survived, but neither do earthquakes figure prominently in any of these. This stands in contrast to the legends of Pacific Northwest tribes, which describe large-scale upheavals of land and sea consistent with the expected results of great earthquakes. Perhaps this reflects a difference in the timing of great earthquakes in both regions. That is, the penultimate great Owens Valley earthquake might have happened far earlier than the 1700 Cascadia event, and therefore slipped further from collective memory by the time European settlers arrived. But legends can certainly have roots that reach back more than a few hundred years; perhaps earthquakes in the Owens Valley simply had a less profound cultural influence than great Cascadia earthquakes. As is often noted, earthquakes don't kill people; buildings kill people. Even a large temblor may have little lasting effect on people who live in light, temporary structures—as long as they are not in the path of rock avalanches. In Cascadia, however, the immense and manifest effects of large-scale uplift and subsidence, as well as tsunamis, could scarcely fail to leave a lasting impression.

With such fragmentary knowledge of the Paiute peoples, such musings clearly remain in the realm of speculation. And time marches on, for better or for worse. Native tribes gave way to miners who in turn gave way to ranchers. Before the local water supply was tapped (many would say pirated) to fill the growing water demands of southern California, the valley was home to thriving farms and orchards. In more recent times, the Owens Valley has supported a range of endeavors, including ranching and, increasingly, outdoor-oriented tourism. At just under 15,000 feet, Mount Whitney, the highest peak in the contiguous United States, attracts a steady stream of intrepid hikers. The less adventurous flock to the scenic Whitney Portal and to the ancient bristlecone pines high in the White Mountains on the east side of the valley, among other destinations.

The grandeur of the Sierra Nevada geographically defines the Owens Valley to the west and the more gentle but still formidable White Mountains and Inyo Mountains define it to the east. Episodes of volcanic activity have shaped the

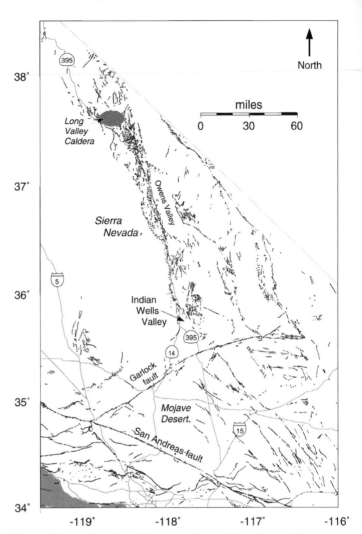

The Mojave Desert and Owens Valley regions

valley throughout its past. This setting makes it at least as dynamic and wonderfully complex as any other part of the California plate-boundary system.

The overall framework of the Owens Valley has less to do with the modern plate boundary and everything to do with processes that were active many million years ago. Until about 30 million years before present, subduction of oceanic crust offshore led to the creation of mountains onshore. According to one modern theory, mountain building is a consequence of compression, or squeezing, across a subduction zone. Some of this compression drives subduction, but some of it is transmitted through to the continent, pushing mountains and plateaus upward.

Once subduction ceases, the raised terrain begins to subside, a complex process whereby some lifted blocks tilt while others subside. The Sierra Nevada tilted westward, creating relatively gentle topography along its western front and more stark and jagged topography to the east. Part of the overall subsidence also led to the formation of the Owens Valley, a so-called rift valley between upward-tilting blocks. The Owens Valley exhibits many of the features typical of rift valleys, including abundant volcanism and geothermal activity. It would not do justice to this chapter of the California story to merely find fault in the Owens Valley. To understand and appreciate this area, we must find volcanoes as well.

But first, the faults.

Owens Valley Faults, Big and Small

As we've already seen, individual faults end, but fault systems commonly feed into other fault systems, particularly systems of strike-slip faults. Think of it as a space issue. Rocks cannot compress, and they have limited ability to warp, or deform, in a gradual fashion. So if one big block of crust moves laterally with respect to the other side of a fault, it invariably represents a "push" or "pull" force that affects the crust at either end of the fault. Consider now the Mojave Desert faults, discussed in chapter 6, which generally accommodate right-lateral motion. This motion will not necessarily transfer beyond the Garlock fault if the blocks within the Mojave experience substantial long-term rotation. Geologic evidence shows that the blocks do indeed undergo such rotation. Nevertheless, the plate boundary does not stop at the Garlock fault. Some of the shearing in the Mojave continues farther northward.

Things soon get complicated, however, once we cross the Garlock fault. Along U.S. 395, we cross the Garlock fault just after passing through the small town of Johannesburg, which was named around 1897 after the famous South African mining town. The fault crosses the road about 3 miles north of the turnoff to the historic mining town of Randsburg, a side excursion well worth the mile drive from the highway. Beyond the turnoff, the fault runs along the base of the El Paso Mountains, crossing the highway at a right angle.

The 150-mile-long Garlock fault is itself a complex zone. Although primarily a left-lateral strike-slip fault, the zone includes the El Paso fault, a steeply dipping structure that accommodates normal—that is, vertical—motion. West of U.S. 395, California 14 crosses the Garlock fault system 2.9 miles north of the Randsburg Road turnoff, just as the highway bends west into Red Rock Canyon. Here, springs along the fault zone generate a constant seeping, feeding streams that are visible from the highway.

Just south of Red Rock Canyon, we turn east onto Redrock-Randsburg Road, which parallels the Garlock fault. Along this lonely stretch of roadway, the main trace of the fault is to the north, along the base of the hills. Driving east we reach a fork in the road, where we continue on Redrock-Randsburg Road toward the south-southeast, passing through Randsburg. Bearing east-northeast from the fork, Garlock Road continues to run just south of the fault until we hit U.S. 395. The main fault trace lies about a mile north of the junction between Garlock Road and U.S. 395.

After climbing over the El Paso Mountains on U.S. 395, we drop into the Indian Wells Valley, something of a little brother to the larger Owens Valley that lies to its immediate north. U.S. 395 skirts around the town of Ridgecrest, which grew up around a navy base in China Lake. Established in the 1940s at the site of a dry lake, China Lake has served as the navy's primary weapons development and testing laboratory for more than half a century. A turnoff from U.S. 395 at the southern end of the Indian Wells Valley leads directly into Ridgecrest (a desert community that seemed like the middle of nowhere to me when, as a child in the 1960s and 1970s, I would visit my grandparents' house there).

But if the Indian Wells Valley seems duller than, well, dirt to an east-coast ten year old with other ideas about appealing attractions in southern California, it has vastly more charms for a person with properly mature—and geologic—sensibilities.

Ridgecrest is not, as one might imagine, on the top of a ridge, but rather toward the eastern edge of the Indian Wells Valley. The town's name owes its existence to the U.S. Post Office, which balked at the more logical first choice, Sierra View, that citizens of the nascent civilian town next to the base proposed. Post office officials vetoed the name because of the abundance of towns with similar and potentially confusing names. Of the names batted around among local residents, Ridgecrest emerged as the consensus choice.

But I digress. In recent times, earthquake activity in the Ridgecrest region has been centered primarily on a shatter pattern of right-lateral fault segments that accommodate right-lateral shearing transferred from the Mojave. Geologists have identified numerous small fault segments in this region: in map view they convey an impression of shattered glass, although they are generally aligned north-south. On August 17, 1995, one of these segments sprang to life with the M5.4 Ridgecrest earthquake. The quake fortunately struck about 6 miles (10 kilometers) north of the town and caused little more than anxiety. Longtime residents of Ridgecrest are no strangers to the power of large earthquakes, as inhabitants in this region strongly felt both the 1952 Kern County earthquake (see chapter 6) and the 1992 Landers earthquake. Two other moderate earthquakes, a M5.8 on September 20, 1995, and a M5.4 on January 7, 1996, followed the first event in 1995.

The recent Ridgecrest activity occurred within a restricted part of the navy base—a bombing range, to be precise. In this case, however, there is little to see. None of the ruptures reached the surface or caused more than very minor surface cracking, the signs of which storms and shifting sands have long since erased.

In general, the Indian Wells Valley represents something of an enigma. It is not clear if the jumble of fault segments that was active in 1995–96 includes faults that are large enough to rupture in M7.0+ earthquakes. Yet it doesn't seem

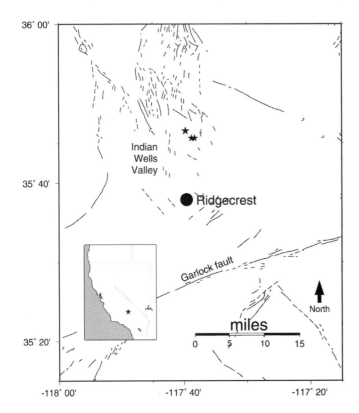

Mapped faults in the Indian Wells Valley and locations (indicated as stars) of primary events during the 1995–96 Ridgecrest sequence

possible that one could have M7.0+ earthquakes south (in Landers) and north (in the Owens Valley) but only a smattering of moderate earthquakes in between. Somehow, at some time, the middle must catch up to the ends.

The recent InSAR results discussed in chapter 6, which show that strain is now accumulating along a line that continues across the Garlock fault into the Indian Wells Valley, might provide a clue to how this catching up will eventually happen. If an earthquake—or series of earthquakes, like the 1992 Joshua Tree–Landers sequence—eventually does rupture a northwest-trending fault that crosses the Garlock fault, finding faults in the Indian Wells Valley will be a far easier endeavor than it is at present. However, such a temblor would likely hit desert communities such as Ridgecrest very hard. Were the strain to be released in a single event, a 75-mile (120-kilometer) rupture would likely produce an earthquake close to M7.5, although an event of this magnitude might not be possible given the apparent lack of a single, through-going fault that spans the zone.

Leaving Ridgecrest for points north along U.S. 395, we soon arrive at a turn-off for a site known as Fossil Falls. Although it has nothing to do with faults, this stop is worthwhile for any student—amateur or professional—of planet Earth. The origin of the falls dates back approximately 10,000 years, when lava from the Coso field to the north flowed southward and eventually crossed the path

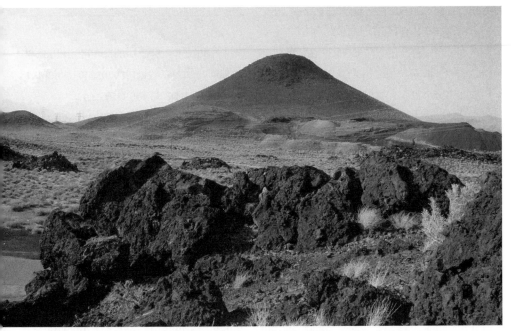

The red cinder cone that rises just east of U.S. 395, north of Ridgecrest (35 58.63N, 117 55.27W)

of an Ice Age river. In time, the river cut a path through the lava flow and polished the black basalt into smoothly rounded contours. When the post-Ice Age climate warmed and dried, the river dried up, leaving behind Fossil Falls.

The Fossil Falls area became more arid gradually. For thousands of years it was home to Paiute peoples, whose handiwork is still preserved as smooth grinding holes in the basalt and small chips of obsidian scattered on the desert floor. (Any and all artifacts are protected by law, and must be left undisturbed.) Obsidian chips at Fossil Falls are by definition artifacts, because the shiny volcanic glass never existed naturally in this particular region. Most of the obsidian remnants are the detritus of anthropologic activity on the part of native tribes—perhaps the state's earliest miners—who exported obsidian from Coso, several miles north of Fossil Falls.

The water and game that once supported native tribes are long gone, but the complex morphology of the falls remains to be explored and appreciated. Furthermore, the ability of the falls to support life has not been fully exhausted. In spring, they come alive with an array of desert wildflowers and, remarkably, with brine shrimp, whose larvae survive in a dormant state through long months of searing heat.

Coso, the volcanic wellspring of the Fossil Falls rocks, lies not far to the north. Between Fossil Falls and Coso, we pass another impressive volcanic feature, a prominent red cinder cone just east of U.S. 395. Known as Red Cinder Cone, it

Writing on the Wall

California's petroglyphs raise an obvious question: In cultures that have no conventional tradition of inscribing words or letters, why write on the walls?

Clearly rock art represented a complex form of expression. The practice is thought to have been carried out largely by shamans, the traditional medicine men who communed with supernatural powers. The tradition of the shaman's trance, induced by natural hallucinogens such as native tobacco, is also well established.

Considering the locations of petroglyph sites in California, the seismologist cannot help but notice that many, if not most, of these sites are in seismically active regions. Is it possible that California's earliest inhabitants left writing on the walls in response to California's earliest historic earthquakes?

That we find rock art near faults is not surprising; as a rule, rocks in California are found near faults. Still, consider some of the best-known petroglyph sites. Rock art sites are so abundant in the seismically active Superstition Wilderness area that some scholars have made the (now discredited) suggestion that native peoples in this region simply had an abundance of free time. The Coso area, which boasts one of the biggest concentrations of rock art anywhere in California, is similarly well known for earthquake (and volcanic) activity.

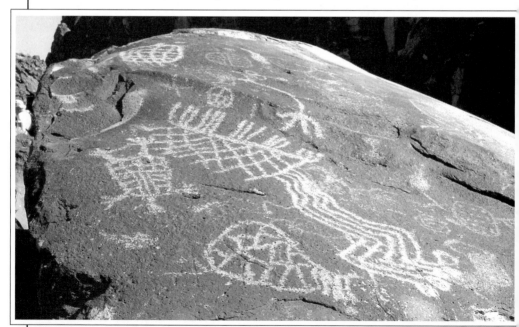

Petroglyphs in Little Petroglyph Canyon, near the Coso geothermal site. Anthropologists commonly interpret wavy lines, which are common here, within these figures as symbols of snakes or serpents. Surviving oral legends of Native American tribes associate snakes and serpents with unrest within the earth. The central petroglyph here is especially suggestive of volcanic activity.

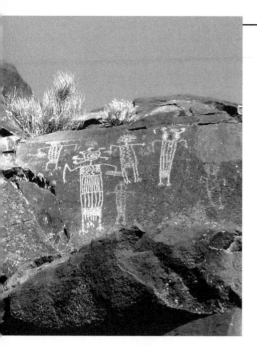

Petroglyphs of shaman figures in Little Petroglyph Canyon. The wavy lines may imply unrest within the earth.

Scientists are wary of the all-too-familiar pitfall of observing a correspondence between two phenomena and linking them as cause and effect. To argue for a causal relationship, we need evidence beyond a simple correspondence.

Perhaps such evidence exists in modern echoes. Earthquake-related legends do not abound among the oral histories of California tribes, but we can find some suggestive hints. The legends of the Agua Caliente Indians describe Tahquitz Canyon, just south of Mount San Jacinto, as the home of the spiritual being Tahquitz. According to legend, the seismic rumbling sometimes heard in the canyon is the growling of the malevolent Tahquitz.

Tahquitz Canyon is considered an especially sacred site even in modern times. Access is restricted, but tribal guides lead visitors on hikes to view the canyon, its spectacular 60-foot waterfall, and its ancient rock art. Tahquitz is near downtown Palm Springs, a stone's throw (so to speak) away from the San Andreas fault. The canyon cuts into hard rock at the base of Mount San Jacinto. Earthquake waves arriving from the south, for example from the highly active San Jacinto fault, would travel very efficiently through the mountain. Temblors would likely be felt and even heard in or near Tahquitz Canyon.

The Southern Diegueno tribe tell similar legends. The Superstition Mountains feature prominently in their oral traditions, and the very name of the mountains reportedly is tied to an earthquake that struck during a ceremony by ancient tribal members. Other legends describe moans and terrible sounds emanating from the caverns at the base of the mountains.

Considering the extent to which earthquakes are etched into the collective psyche of present-day Californians, perhaps it would only be surprising if the surviving written expressions of the state's earliest human inhabitants did not reflect the region's tumultuous natural environment. California has always been Earthquake Country; Californians have always found, and will always find, ways to come to grips with this.

is the iron-rich remnant of a long-dead minor volcano. This cone was not, however, the source of the lava flows that formed Fossil Falls.

Coso is a volcanic region that, to this day, remains active. In the 1930s and 1940s, the Coso geothermal field was open to the public and was also the site of a resort spa known for its rejuvenative mineral waters. Waters from the site were bottled and sold; mud was scooped up by hand and packed into jars. Coso's resort days ended in the early 1940s when the U.S. Navy acquired the land. Some remnants of the resort facilities remain, thoroughly battered by the ravages of time and increased geothermal activity.

In the heart of the Coso region, we find boiling mud pots, thermal springs, and other dramatic features of geothermal activity—in addition to the vast engineering technology built to exploit the natural power source. Today Coso is home to an active geothermal energy production field jointly owned and operated by the U.S. Navy and private industry. It also lies behind locked gates, inaccessible to anyone who does not have official business there. But fear not: there are accessible and equally dramatic volcanic and geothermal features yet to come.

The Coso region makes its presence felt, if not seen because the ongoing volcanic activity drives an especially high level of earthquake activity. The rate of felt earthquakes—M3.0 and up—in the Coso area is among the highest found in the state. At this point, we might stop to consider whether it is a coincidence that this area is also one of the most spectacular petroglyph sites in California.

Leaving the falls behind and passing Coso, we quickly approach a stretch of U.S. 395 from which we can (at long last) find a fault: the Owens Valley fault, which ruptured in 1872, producing an earthquake estimated at M7.6. This fault runs along the base of the Sierra Nevada not far west of the highway. The 1872 rupture involved primarily strike-slip motion, but also a big enough component of normal motion to leave behind a conspicuous fault scarp. From U.S. 395 around the small town of Olancha, the scarp starts to be visible as a stair-step offset running along the base of the hills.

The best place to find this fault, however, is near the town that bore the brunt of the earthquake's fury. In 1872, the mining community of Lone Pine included fifty-nine buildings, most of adobe construction, and a few hundred residents. The temblor struck at 2:30 A.M. on March 26 and generated perceptible ground motions from Mexico to Canada. Near ground zero along the Owens Valley fault, many simple masonry homes were quickly reduced to rubble, claiming at least twenty-seven lives and leaving only seven buildings standing in Lone Pine. The quake caused significant damage throughout the Owens Valley. In Independence, about 15 miles (25 kilometers) north of Lone Pine, the county courthouse collapsed. The earthquake triggered massive landslides along the Sierra Nevada and permanently altered the flow of groundwater in many areas.

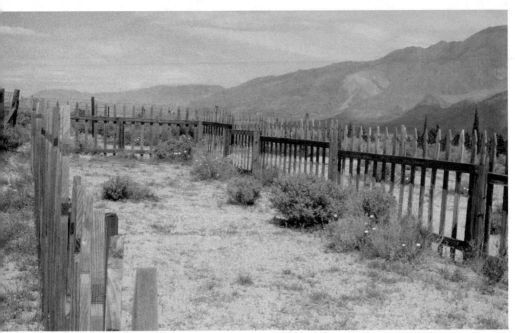

Mass gravesite of sixteen victims of the 1872 Lone Pine earthquake, just north of the town of Lone Pine (36 37.11N, 118 04.13W)

During winter of 1872, famed naturalist John Muir was employed as a caretaker of Black's Hotel on the west side of the Sierra. Revealing himself to be a true scholar of the earth, Muir later wrote, "Though I had never before enjoyed a storm of this sort, the strange, wild, thrilling motion and rumbling could not be mistaken, and I ran out of my cabin, near the Sentinel Rock, both glad and frightened, shouting, 'A noble earthquake!' feeling sure I was going to learn something." Muir went on to describe a cascade of boulders into the valley, and a "free curve luminous from friction, making a terribly sublime and beautiful spectacle—an arc of fire fifteen hundred feet span, as true in form and as steady as a rainbow, in the midst of the stupendous roaring rock storm." Such lights were observed along the eastern Sierra Nevada as well, where the shaking released innumerable rockfalls.

After two months of aftershocks and subsequent avalanches, Muir surveyed the changed landscape with approval. Looking back he summed up his feeling about the experience—and in so doing revealed the essence of the naturalist's soul: "Storms of every sort, torrents, earthquakes, cataclysms, 'convulsions of nature,' etc., however mysterious and lawless at first sight they may seem, are only harmonious notes in the song of creation, varied expressions of God's love."

It is fair to note, however, that Muir "enjoyed" the earthquake at a fairly safe distance; he did not have a front row seat to the degree of lawlessness associated with the powerful temblor closer to its source. Evidence of such lawlessness can still be found in the Lone Pine area today. At a turnoff just north of the charming

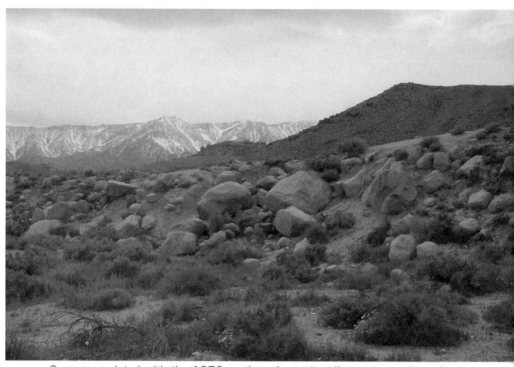

Scarp associated with the 1872 earthquake and earlier ruptures along the Owens Valley fault (36 36.33N 118 04.50W)

modern town, we arrive at one of the most poignant stops on an earthquake tour of the state: a weathered wooden picket fence enclosing the mass grave of sixteen of the earthquake's victims. Sixteen men, women, and children, each accorded perhaps three or four feet of lateral space. Standing at one end, with gentle breezes swirling overhead, one cannot help being moved by the expanse of ground within the fence perimeter. Appropriately enough, during the spring wildflower season the earth summons forth blazing yellow desert dandelions to grace this otherwise most spartan of gravesites. The scarp associated with the 1872 earthquake can be seen to the southwest of the gravesite, a seemingly gentle ribbon of offset along the base of the hills.

Returning to U.S. 395 and Lone Pine, we can head west on Whitney Portal Road, which, as its name suggests, makes a winding ascent before coming to an end at the Whitney Portal. A mere 0.9 mile from U.S. 395, we find a fault—the scarp of the 1872 rupture. After turning west onto Whitney Portal Road, proceed for 0.6 mile to a dirt road just before the aqueduct. Turn right onto the dirt road and bear right following the trees after 0.2 mile. Approximately 0.3 mile beyond the trees, we arrive at the fault scarp. Scientists have investigated this scarp in detail and think it is the result of three separate earthquakes over 10,000 years.

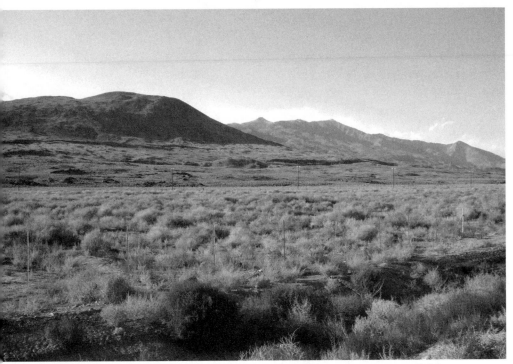

Two segments of the fault scarp created by the 1872 earthquake are visible from U.S. 395 approximately 20 miles north of Independence. (37 6.09N, 118 15.11W)

Together they caused approximately 22 feet (7 meters) of vertical offset and fully 55 feet (17 meters) of right-lateral offset. The 1872 temblor alone accounted for more than 3 feet of vertical movement and nearly 19 feet (6 meters) of lateral motion. The 1872 rupture extended many miles beyond Lone Pine, reaching nearly to Bishop, and is still evident from many points along U.S. 395 as we head north away from the town. The scarp is particularly clear between 20 and 25 miles north of Independence, again to the west of the highway.

As we head north from Lone Pine, we are reminded that the Owens Valley is home to more than geologic points of interest. Twelve miles north of Lone Pine, we arrive at the turnoff for Manzanar, the wartime internment camp established in 1942 to detain Japanese-Americans whom the U.S. government considered a national security threat. Before the war, Manzanar was home to thriving apple and pear orchards. At its peak as an internment camp, the population of Manzanar swelled to 10,000, the largest settlement in the history of the Owens Valley. Little remains of the once-substantial complex except a few fragments of structures, and perhaps the ghostly echoes from an unhappy chapter in American history.

A few miles north of Manzanar we can find more—and more benign—history in the town of Independence, the county seat of Inyo County. The Eastern California

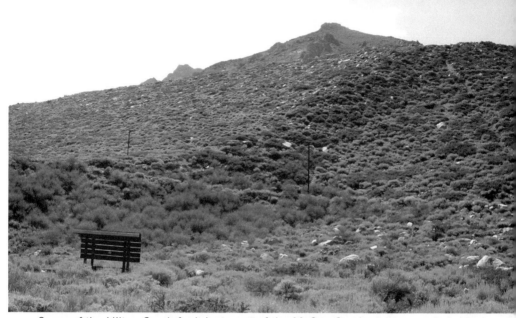

Scarp of the Hilton Creek fault just west of the McGee Creek campground and just south of Long Valley Caldera (37 33.86N 118 47.16W)

Museum features Paiute artifacts as well as artifacts from the region's mining days. The Edwards House, constructed in 1863, just two years after the first permanent habitation of any sort was built in the Owens Valley, is the oldest building in the region—a rare and noble survivor of the 1872 temblor. The county courthouse dates back to 1923, built after its first three predecessors succumbed to the earthquake, a fire, and the winds of change, respectively.

Heading north away from Independence, we pass another red cinder cone, Crater Mountain, which rises west of the highway about 36 miles north of Lone Pine. Crater Mountain is one of thirty-odd cones in the Taboose–Big Pine volcanic field, which had four separate eruptive episodes about 200,000 years ago.

North of Bishop on U.S. 395, we begin to climb Sherwin Grade, which leads into an area whose geography and topography were created by an enormous volcanic eruption in Long Valley about 760,000 years ago. That eruption spewed the Bishop tuff, an enormous formation of mostly hardened volcanic ash that thickly blankets the landscape southeast of Long Valley. As we climb toward the caldera, the desert gives way to mountainous terrain with more trees, a more temperate summer, and a much colder winter.

A few miles beyond the small community of Tom's Place, we arrive at the turnoff for McGee Creek Road, which leads to the McGee Creek campground after about 2 miles. Along the hill immediately west of the campground, we can see a subtle but characteristic slope break: the Hilton Creek fault. The Hilton Creek fault can also be seen from U.S. 395 at the turnoff for McGee Creek. This fault, although seemingly well developed, has played an enigmatic role in recent earthquake activity in the area. Sequences of earthquakes through the 1980s and 1990s popped off all around the Hilton Creek fault, but many of them were on secondary faults in the area.

At the McGee Creek campground, there is another notable earthquake site, although it might not look like one at first glance: a very large boulder just beyond the nominal perimeter of a campsite on the north side of the campground. Until June 1998, this boulder was perched on the hillside above the campground on the scarp of the Hilton Creek fault. The M5.1 earthquake in June 1998 dislodged the massive rock, which tumbled down the hill. Most fortunately, it came to rest before reaching any inhabited campsites, but the huge tumbling rock carved a track in the hillside that has remained visible for years.

Like the episodes of unrest that preceded it, the 1998 sequence of quakes died away with a whimper, not a bang, leaving scientists to once again bide their time until the mercurial caldera system springs to life again. After leaving the McGee Creek campground, our next stop is the Big Kahuna of California volcanoes: Long Valley Caldera.

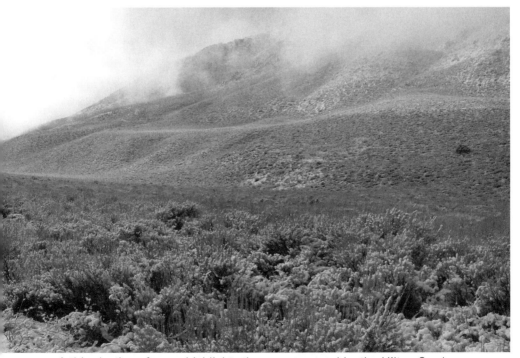

A thin dusting of snow highlights the groove carved by the Hilton Creek fault in the hillside just west of U.S. 395 near the McGee Creek turnoff. (37 34.81N, 118 47.31W)

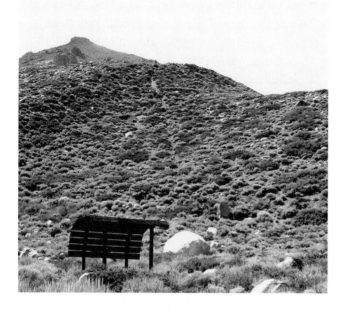

A M5.1 earthquake in 1998 jostled loose the large whitish boulder, which tumbled down the hill to its resting place just north of a campsite within the McGee Creek campground. The track the boulder left was still clearly visible when this photograph was taken, four years later. (37 33.86N 118 47.16W)

Long Valley: A Restless Caldera

South of Bishop, the Owens Valley/U.S. 395 corridor has, like most of the rest of California, been shaped by plate motions past and present—which is to say, it has been shaped by its faults. Once we arrive at Bishop, however, and begin the climb up and into Long Valley Caldera, finding faults is largely beside the point. At least, it is if the point is to understand the geologic forces that have shaped the landscape.

To be sure, Long Valley has experienced its share of earthquakes in recent decades, the vast majority of them indistinguishable from earthquakes anywhere else. That is, they rupture on garden-variety faults in response to local and/or regional forces. So, like the rest of California, Long Valley does have its faults. But to understand what makes this part of California tick (and possibly explode), we have to understand what drives the faults.

Since 1980, earthquake activity clearly related to volcanic activity at Long Valley has been scattered over different locations both inside and outside of the caldera. The interplay between volcanoes and faults is complex, and we will examine that relationship at more length later in this chapter. The two processes are intertwined, and we are left with a fundamental chicken-and-egg quandary: Is there volcanic activity at Long Valley because tectonic forces are opening the door for magma to rise to the surface, or is the magma providing the fundamental regional impetus driving the faulting processes?

If the question seems perplexing, rest assured that professional earth scientists grapple with it as well. The answer may be that chickens and eggs have to be considered on several different scales. On a large scale, geologist Tanya Atwater has observed that the Sierra Nevada north of Long Valley is rotating counterclockwise while to the south it is rotating clockwise. This may explain why a long-lived zone of crustal extension exists at the hinge point—Long Valley. Alternatively, others have suggested that the volcanic activity at Long Valley is the result of the death throes of subduction along the coast. According to the so-called slabless-window hypothesis, continental crust in the Long Valley area was underlaid not by a sinking slab of oceanic crust but by hot mantle rock. Although markedly different, both hypotheses suggest that large-scale plate-tectonic forces fundamentally drive the volcanic activity at Long Valley.

Whatever the true explanation, within the larger tectonic framework there is evidence that magmatic activity drives local seismic activity. Specifically, measurements of ground deformation, which track movement of underground magma, show that events of magma intrusion precede episodes of seismic unrest. So while the volcanic system might be there because of large-scale plate-tectonic motions and forces, most of the ongoing earthquakes appear to be the result of volcanic unrest.

When magma deep underground moves, it pushes the ground upward, and the crust crackles in response. "Crackle" is a good word for it: Rising magma, be it in blobs or thin blades called dikes, generates a complex pattern of stress in the surrounding crust and a complicated, crackly pattern of faults. Finding faults in Long Valley Caldera tends not to be fruitful because the faults are myriad and complex. Finding volcanic features, however, is another matter. Thus will we embark on a detour of our fault-finding adventures to focus on a tour of this remarkable volcanic region.

To set the stage for the tour, it will help to understand the volcanic history and setting of Long Valley. For this we might first need to adjust our ideas about volcanoes. Well-known Cascadia volcanoes such as Mount Saint Helens and Mount Rainier match stereotypes of the type of volcanoes known to blow their tops in movies. But throughout earth's history, the most cataclysmic eruptions have been of a different scale altogether, and some of them left behind enormous calderas. We can barely appreciate the full scale of Long Valley Caldera from ground level, as it stretches some 20 miles (30 kilometers) east to west. From ground level, the perimeter of the caldera is far from obvious in many places—especially to the east, where no clear caldera rim exists. Where U.S. 395 crosses the southeast rim of the caldera just after skirting around the southwest side of Lake Crowley, the caldera rim is decidedly subtle.

Scientists have painstakingly assembled the history of eruptive activity at Long Valley through decades of geologic investigations aimed at identifying different types of volcanic rock and, using modern dating techniques, obtaining reliable

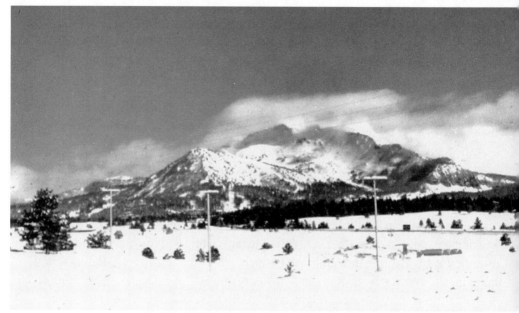
Mammoth Mountain

estimates of their ages. The work is a little like dissecting a stale layer cake, one messy—and hard—rock layer at a time.

The oldest volcanic layer in Long Valley is more of a blob than a layer. Glass Mountain, a relatively small dome on the east side of the caldera, resulted from eruptions between about 1 million and 800,000 years before present. The really big bang at Long Valley happened fairly soon (in geologic terms) after the Glass Mountain eruptions. The truly massive, caldera-forming eruption of Long Valley blew around 760,000 years before present. Whereas the 1980 eruption of Mount Saint Helens in Washington involved a crater about 1 mile (2 kilometers) across and spewed about 0.05 cubic mile (0.25 cubic kilometer) of total ejected material, the Long Valley eruption involved a caldera some 20 miles (30 kilometers) long, with some 130 cubic miles (600 cubic kilometers) of erupted material. Picture an eruption like the one the world witnessed in 1980—but 2,400 times larger. Ash from Long Valley drifted around the world. The ash cloud spread out over much of what is now the western United States, reaching as far east as present-day Nebraska.

On a local scale, the most dramatic signature of the Long Valley eruption, aside from the caldera itself, is known as the Bishop tuff, a large, thick blanket of consolidated volcanic ash that covers many square miles around Long Valley. This rock is the fossilized evidence of the so-called pyroclastic flow, one of the most locally hazardous components of eruptions such as Mount Saint Helens and Long Valley. Such a flow consists of a massive, very hot cloud of pulverized rock suspended in volcanic gases. Set into motion when a big eruption begins, the huge cloud barrels down the mountainside at speeds of about 100 miles per hour, flattening everything in its path.

Geologists have mapped and studied the Bishop tuff in great detail. One of the most impressive fossil pyroclastic flows on the planet, it provides important clues into the detailed eruption sequence of Long Valley. Massive caldera-forming eruptions on a scale of Long Valley happen anywhere on earth no more than perhaps once every 100,000 years. That is fortunate for us, as such an event would not only devastate the local and regional environs but also change the climate worldwide. Since 760,000 years before present, volcanic activity at Long Valley has continued at a far less apocalyptic, and far more typical, pace.

Geologic investigations reveal a burst of activity around 100,000 years ago, including the beginning of a series of eruptions on the western edge of Long Valley Caldera. Over the next 50,000 or so years, these so-called dome-building eruptions produced Mammoth Mountain. Just east of the turnoff to Mammoth, the Casa Diablo Geothermal Power Plant hums steadily, drawing hot water (334 degrees Fahrenheit!) from depths of 600 feet to produce electricity that supplies one-third to one-fourth of the power for the town of Mammoth Lakes. Although tucked out of view from the highway, in winter the area around the plant often stands out like a sore—or rather a brown—thumb, its warmed ground free of the snow that typically blankets the rest of the caldera.

We'll explore the Mammoth Lakes region in more detail shortly, but for now we'll pick up our tour farther north along U.S. 395. The most recent volcanic activity at Long Valley has taken place along a north-south line that begins just north of Mammoth Mountain and heads north, more or less along U.S. 395, to Mono Lake. This series of eruptions generally left behind classic volcanic craters and domes, leading to a string of volcanic features known as the Mono-Inyo chain of craters. Evidence suggests that activity migrated northward along this chain over the course of the last few thousand years, and that the most recent eruption occurred in the middle of Mono Lake about 250 years ago.

The geology of the Mono-Inyo chain tells us that the recent eruptions had a grab bag of styles: a few of them were primarily lava flows, such as we now find on Hawaii; others were more explosive. It appears, however, that all of them resulted from a blade, or dike, of fairly soupy magma that traveled west and north from a magma source under the central caldera. (Geologists classify three primary, types of magma that correspond with the acronym BAD: basalt, the least viscous or most soupy; andesite, intermediate in viscosity; and dacite, the thickest, least soupy type.) One speculation has been that the caldera-forming eruption essentially blocked the direct upward conduit for magma, forcing it to squirt sideways.

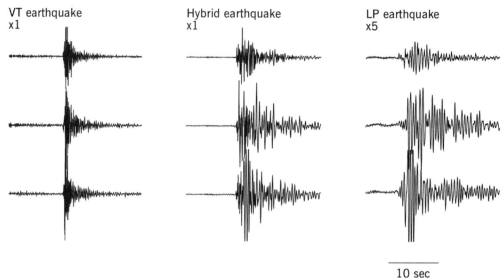

VT earthquake
x1

Hybrid earthquake
x1

LP earthquake
x5

10 sec

Seismograms from a typical earthquake *(left)* compared to the
recording of a so-called long-period earthquake *(right),* which
was generated not by motion on faults but by the movement of underground fluid.
Seismologists also commonly observe so-called hybrid events *(middle)* in volcanic
regions, and they think the events reflect a combined process of fluid motion and
faulting. Long-period earthquakes do not last longer than typical earthquakes, but their
vibrations contain longer-period energy—that is, the period of time required for one
up-and-down swing is longer than for a typical earthquake of the same magnitude.
—DATA FROM THE MONTESSERAT VOLCANO OBSERVATORY

The question is, what's next? Substantial magma still lurks beneath the bucolic
surface at Long Valley—perhaps as a central, coherent magma chamber or perhaps as more of a raisin bread of magma blobs. Three lines of evidence provide
incontrovertible evidence for the presence of magma at depth. First, the middle
part of the caldera, the so-called resurgent dome, has been rising since at least
1980, pushed upward by a magma source estimated to be at a depth of 4 miles
(6 to 7 kilometers). Second, gas, primarily carbon dioxide, vents from the surface
at many places around the caldera, suggesting that upwardly migrating magma
either ruptured sealed pockets of gas deep in the crust or that dissolved gasses
within the magma escaped as the molten rock reached more shallow depths. And
third, since 1989 seismologists have observed a characteristic type of earthquake
known as a long-period event, which results from the underground movement
of magma or magmatic fluids, as opposed to slip on a fault. Unlike other types
of seismic signals that volcanoes generate (see chapter 8), long-period earthquakes
are not harbingers of imminent eruption. They do, however, let us know in no
uncertain terms that magma is moving around down there.

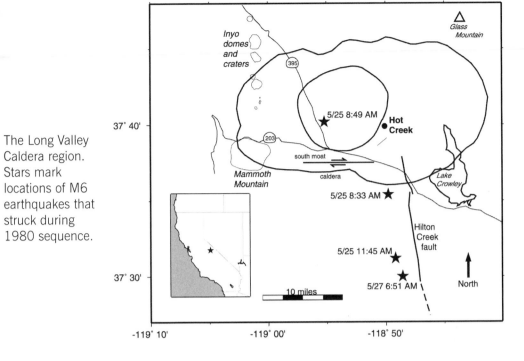

The Long Valley Caldera region. Stars mark locations of M6 earthquakes that struck during 1980 sequence.

According to seismic and other evidence, the current episode of unrest began with a whimper, relatively speaking, in the late 1970s. After producing few felt earthquakes for the previous decades, a M5.8 earthquake struck just east of Long Valley Caldera in 1978. The whimper turned to a bang on May 25, 1980, just a week after Mount Saint Helens erupted, when a M6 earthquake hit south of the caldera. Two more earthquakes of similar magnitude struck before the day was over, including one within the caldera. Two days later, a fourth earthquake, of about the same size, hit.

With the attention of both the public and most volcano scientists focused northward, the 1980s rumblings at Long Valley generated muted excitement. However, they did not escape the attention of scientists, including David Hill of the U.S. Geological Survey, who, although he didn't know it at the time, was at the beginning of a twenty-year odyssey that would prove at least as challenging politically as scientifically.

Magmatic activity caused the burst of earthquakes in 1980. Later investigations showed that the resurgent dome rose about 10 inches (25 centimeters) during the episode. The region did settle down, however, and both uplift and earthquake activity tapered off sharply.

Long Valley continued to percolate after 1980, but at a more subdued level. When a number of moderate earthquakes struck in early 1982, scientists at the U.S. Geological Survey recommended that a "watch" be issued in light of concerns

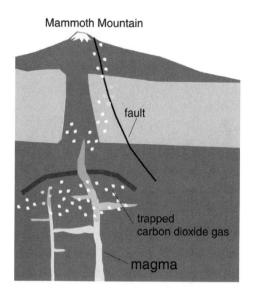

Mammoth Mountain

fault

trapped
carbon dioxide gas

magma

The inferred nature of the volcanic system beneath Mammoth Mountain. In 1989, magma rising deep beneath the mountain apparently broke through a seal *(the curved gray line)* that had trapped gasses, primarily carbon dioxide, underground. The gas then migrated upward, following faults to reach the surface on the flanks of the mountain.

for future activity. At that time, a watch was considered one step below a warning, which would have been issued had there been signs of an imminent eruption. State officials considered the evidence and drafted a "notice of potential hazard." The language of the notice was carefully crafted to avoid any hint that an eruption might be imminent.

Before any statement could be released to the public, however, an article describing the action appeared in the *Los Angeles Times.* Immediately, resorts in Mammoth Lakes, which draw heavily from the greater Los Angeles region, received a flood of cancellations for the upcoming Memorial Day weekend. Thus—especially after the rest of 1982 came and went without any escalation in activity—did the U.S. Geological Survey become persona non grata in the Mammoth Lakes region, a (dubious) distinction that would take years to overcome.

The situation heated up—in more ways than one—when two earthquakes of about M5.0 struck in 1983. The renewed activity punctuated the still-standing watch notice and raised tensions among local leaders. In October of that year, then-Secretary of the Interior James Watt ordered the warning system changed, with the adoption of a single warning level: imminent threat of hazard. This order nullified the standing watch notice that had first alerted the public to a potential hazard in 1982.

Developments over the next few years involved as much politics as science. Two more significant earthquakes shook the region, although centered away from the immediate caldera, in November of 1984 and July of 1986. The latter event, the Chalfant Valley earthquake, registered M6.4 and was widely felt.

In the political arena, the 1986 Challenger disaster preoccupied much of the public's attention. Locally and at high levels within the government, meanwhile,

David Hill in Long Valley

David Hill was at the helm of U.S. Geological Survey monitoring of Long Valley Caldera (the Mammoth Lakes region) through and beyond the 1990s. What the public may not know is that the unrest at Long Valley continued, with fits and starts, for a good twenty years following the burst of earthquakes and underground magma activity in 1980. Through these turbulent years, Hill held primary responsibility for evaluating whether activity reached the criteria for declaring an alert or warning. Activity neared this level in 1989 and again in late 1997.

In November 1997, while evaluating a burst of earthquake activity that had begun the previous summer but escalated alarmingly through the fall, Hill was charged with determining whether the U.S. Geological Survey could comfortably maintain a "green" status (no threat) or whether they should go to "yellow" (some concern). To Hill the activity level appeared vexingly "chartreuse." Mercifully, by December, the activity had begun to show signs of dying down before it crossed the line that would have necessitated an alert.

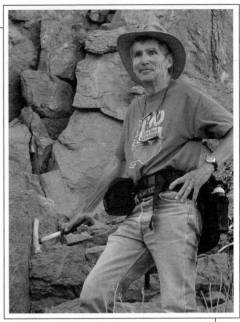

David Hill in the field at Long Valley

The public does not notice, much less applaud, a successful decision to *not* issue an alert or prediction. Yet Hill's decisions to not declare alerts required every bit as much scientific acumen as has gone into the successful predictions of eruptions worldwide in recent years. His decisions were as impressive, and important for the effectiveness and reputation of the U.S. Geological Survey volcano program, as a successful eruption alert would have been.

tensions over Long Valley gave way to a willingness to confront the scientific issues in a more cool-headed manner. Tensions did not, however, disappear entirely, and they certainly did not disappear overnight.

The next significant episode of unrest came in 1989 with a flurry of small earthquakes, this time under Mammoth Mountain itself. By this time, a stepped-up monitoring program of both earthquakes and ground deformation had been in place for more than five years, and scientists were able to show that magma rising beneath Mammoth Mountain had triggered the activity. For the first time, seismologists observed the characteristic long-period events deep under the

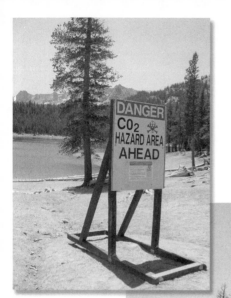

The tree-kill area around Lake Mary. Large warning signs *(top left)* alert visitors to the danger, which has claimed the lives of many trees in the area *(bottom right)*. (37 36.78N 119 01.26W)

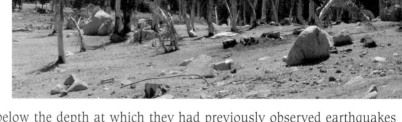

mountain, below the depth at which they had previously observed earthquakes in the area.

Although the magma remained comfortably below the surface, this was the episode that led to a substantial increase in carbon dioxide emissions, which killed trees in substantial numbers across wide areas. Geochemical analysis revealed the gas to have a magmatic origin, and scientists concluded that it had originated at depth and percolated to the surface at a number of locations around the perimeter of the mountain.

Unto itself, carbon dioxide represents a significant hazard for humans, particularly in winter when high concentrations of gas can pond near the ground, under the snow. Concentrations of carbon dioxide in these pockets can be as high as 80 percent, high enough to be fatal to humans in just a few breaths. Warning signs were quickly put up to alert skiers and others to the danger. If you ever come across one, take it seriously.

Once again, the 1989 activity subsided, giving way to a lower level of continued percolation—and continued ambient concern. In the ensuing years, the Department of the Interior, relying on guidance from the U.S. Geological Survey, developed a new system of alerts to replace the single-level warning, culminating in the 1991 development of a five-tiered alphabetic system.

Through the early 1990s, tensions persisted between scientists and local officials, the latter group continuing to have concern over the extent to which the hazard was being exaggerated. But tensions did continue to cool, and during this period town officials worked with scientists to come up with yet another system for alerts, this one based on colors: green (no danger), yellow (some concern), orange (eruption considered imminent), and red (eruption in progress). Scientists developed very detailed scientific criteria as well, which involved an assessment of various types of observations, including earthquake activity and ground deformation.

The new system was put through its paces in 1997, when in February, a M4.0 earthquake struck without further fanfare. But in May and June, data from GPS instruments revealed an episode of uplift beneath the resurgent dome. The earthquakes began in earnest in July. By November, the seismic activity was escalating at a rate high enough to engender real concern among scientists. By this time, monitoring data was available in real time over the Web, so many within the earth-science community watched—and held their breath.

Observed deformation of the ground at Long Valley as measured by GPS instruments through the late 1980s and 1990s. The different curves reflect measurements of deformation along different lines within Long Valley; the top curve corresponds to the rate of uplift of the resurgent dome, the central part of the caldera. The monitoring instruments were not in place in 1980. —U.S. GEOLOGICAL SURVEY DATA

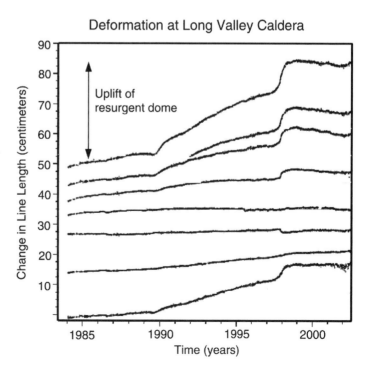

Deformation at Long Valley Caldera

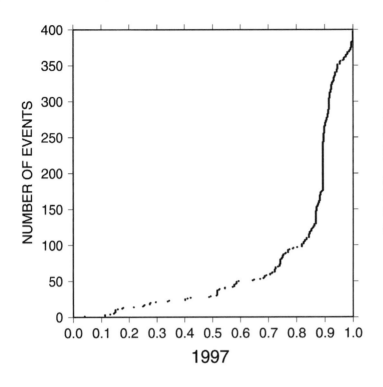

Rate of earthquakes in the Long Valley region through 1997. The rapid escalation of activity in late November came close to the levels at which officials declare alerts.

On November 22, 1997, with the escalation looking more and more worrisome, David Hill of the U.S. Geological Survey and his colleagues were within hours of changing the alert status of the volcano to yellow. But then came the first signs of diminution of the activity, and within days it was clear that, while still active, the episode was tapering off. The anxiety was not entirely over, however, as the region produced a couple of smaller bursts of activity over the next six weeks. Only in early 1998 were scientists able to completely exhale. However, the most energetic earthquake activity was yet to come, a sequence that culminated in the summer of 1998, centered down in the Sierra Block region and judged not to reflect substantial magmatic unrest. This sequence included more than 10,000 reported events, two of M5.1 (the first of which dislodged the McGee Creek boulder we saw earlier). But the sixty-four-thousand-dollar question at Long Valley is, does a sequence directly reflect the movement of magma—and is it, therefore, a possible harbinger of an eruption?

It is perhaps a subtle distinction. Burps and hiccups within the magmatic system at Long Valley appear to drive the earthquake activity. However, some earthquakes are more worrisome than others. Some temblors, such as many of those in the 1989 sequence, are caused directly by magma migrating upwards; other earthquakes result from the shifting of blocks of rock, which can happen well away (in time and space) from moving magma. To distinguish between the two types of events, scientists rely on GPS data to tell us whether the ground is being pushed upward. They also use sophisticated techniques to distinguish between the pattern of waves produced by a standard tectonic earthquake on a fault and those produced directly by moving magma or underground fluid.

While GPS data suggested that migration of underground magma did not accompany the 1998 sequence—which is to say, it was harmless—detailed analysis of seismograms revealed at least a few small earthquakes that did exhibit the characteristic signature of volcanic earthquakes. This, along with a handful of other focused studies over the years, suggests that while the Sierra Block appears to be away from the volcanic action in the central caldera, it may contain a few of the raisins of the raisin-bread magmatic system.

Before leaving this part of the saga, however, we must first take care of unfinished business. What *is* next at Long Valley? The short answer, not surprisingly, is that we don't know. Despite the high level of recent seismic and volcanic activity in the Sierra Block, an eruption in this region would be a substantial departure from the pattern of volcanic activity in the recent geologic past. Considering the timescales over which volcanic systems play out, scientists doubt that we happen to be at a unique cusp that marks a dramatic change in the pattern of eruptions. Perhaps instead we are seeing clues about the future evolution of the enormous volcanic region. Perhaps the past conduits for upward migration of magma are becoming blocked, and faults that are now moving within the Sierra Block will create new conduits. Scientists have shown that magma moving in the central caldera has caused the crust within the Sierra Block to effectively be pulled apart. This process of extension might create conduits along which magma will find its way to the surface—not today and not tomorrow, but some day.

Recent geologic history suggests that the Mono/Inyo chain is the most likely site of the next eruption, which would probably be smaller than the 1980 eruption of Mount Saint Helens. Given the complexity of unrest since 1980, however, we must consider other scenarios, including an eruption on or near Mammoth Mountain, which lies at the southern end of the Mono/Inyo chain, or one within the so-called south moat of the caldera, just south of the resurgent dome. Neither of these, clearly, would be good news from a societal point of view—especially since Mammoth Lakes embarked on a major commercial expansion at the beginning of the twenty-first century.

However, the more benign scenario—a small eruption along the Mono/Inyo chain—remains most likely. And based on historic frequency, researchers have determined the odds of an eruption to be about one in two hundred per year. Perhaps the odds can be considered somewhat higher in light of the recent episode of unrest, but a consideration of similar large, complex caldera systems worldwide reveals that unrest does not always portend disaster. Some calderas, such as Iwo Jima, exhibit substantial activity for decades without blowing their tops.

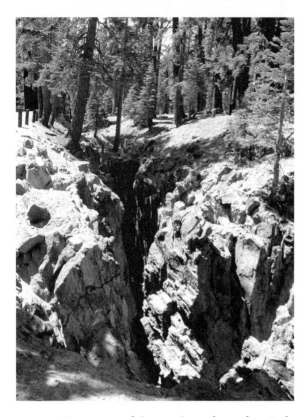

The so-called "Earthquake Fault" on Minaret Road (California 203) between the town of Mammoth Lakes and the main resort area. The absence of lateral offset across this fissure leads most geologists to conclude that it was created by the cooling of volcanic rock rather than by earthquakes. (37 39.22N 119 00.00W)

Upon casual inspection, the volcanic hazard at Long Valley is easy to underestimate, if not to overlook altogether. As noted, the sheer scale of the caldera makes it hard to appreciate from any one vantage point or photograph. Mammoth Mountain looks like the volcano that it is, but it is scarcely *the* volcano—more like a minor pimple on the edge of the massive caldera system. Only in regional maps of topographic relief can we appreciate the full scale of the caldera. Up close, the caldera's contours appear rounded and benign, and we are far more likely to be impressed by the spectacular scenery than by any sense of mortal danger.

Nonetheless, we can certainly find abundant evidence of volcanic unrest if we are inclined to look for it. And so we can return to our tour to explore more of the unique features of Long Valley Caldera. From U.S. 395, California 203 leads into the town of Mammoth Lakes. After 4 miles on California 203, we arrive at an intersection with Lake Mary Road. Veering right on 203 (Minaret Road) and continuing 1.9 miles, we arrive at a sign proclaiming, "Earthquake Fault." Notwithstanding the sign, the origins of this dramatic feature remain enigmatic, as it does not exhibit the usual signs of tectonic faults. Instead, it may represent a mere fissure that opened as part of the cooling process in basalt. The "fault" is worth a stop, in any case.

Continuing along California 203, we eventually reach the central Mammoth Lakes resort facility, from which a shuttle bus ferries passengers down to the

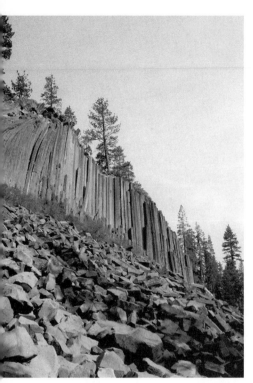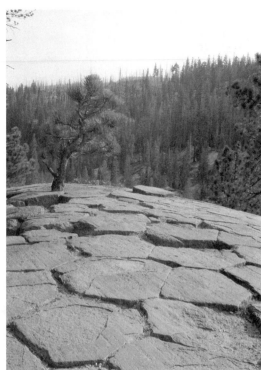

The Devils Postpile is one of the best examples in the world of columnar jointing *(left)*, a hexagonal pattern that forms in basalt as it cools and contracts. Glaciers scoured and gouged these rocks, leaving a smooth surface that, in the view from above *(right),* clearly displays the remarkable regularity of the pattern.

Devils Postpile. The site of volcanic activity thousands of years ago, Devils Postpile is one of the best examples in the world of columnar jointing, the elegant hexagonal pattern that forms in basaltic rocks when they cool under certain conditions. Glaciers exposed the "postpiles" and scoured them clean, gouging linear etchings in the top surface of the basalt as the ice moved over it.

If we return to Lake Mary Road along California 203, turn right, and follow the road for 5.1 miles, we arrive at Horseshoe Lake, site of one of the largest tree-kill areas, which encompassed some 100 acres as of 2002.

We can find one of the most dramatic volcano sites by taking California 203 back to U.S. 395. From the junction, proceed 3 miles to Airport Road and turn right, then turn right onto Fish Hatchery Road after another 0.5 mile. After 1.2 miles, we can see a linear, modest fault scarp—a feature generated during the 1980 earthquake swarm.

But the real attraction lies another 2 miles farther along Fish Hatchery Road: Hot Creek, an area of dramatic, active geothermal activity. A path leads visitors

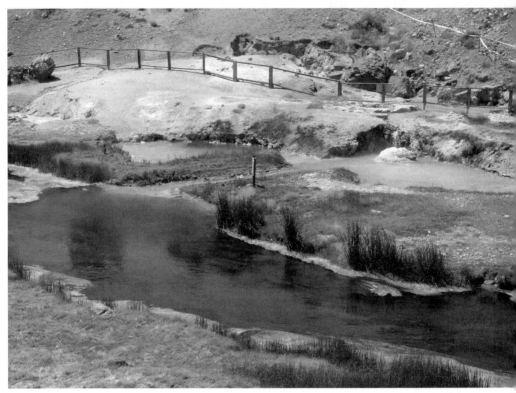

At Hot Creek, north of the Mammoth Lakes airport, geothermal waters burble to the surface. The water's temperature and chemistry create bright turquoise pools *(background)* that provide a stunning contrast to the darker waters of the creek *(foreground)*. (37 39.63N 118 49.67W)

down to view the active fumaroles and hot springs. Along the path, we find ample evidence of where heat and fluids have altered minerals. Typically, altered rock has a chalky and/or bleached appearance. At the main Hot Creek site, we encounter a rainbow: the brownish rocks bleaching to white, the dark to lush green of underwater reeds, the deep blue waters of Hot Creek, and the rich turquoise waters of adjacent geothermal pools. In summer, vibrant orange dragonflies dart above the surface of the creek, embroidering the scene with a splash of warmer hues.

Activity at Hot Creek dates back to 1973, when at least five springs appeared literally overnight on August 24. Two of the springs began as geysers that spouted about 10 feet (3 meters) into the air for several weeks before subsiding and giving way to less violent spring activity. The springs formed within hours of a M3.5 earthquake that centered some 25 miles (40 kilometers) southeast of Hot Creek. While it is possible that shaking from this earthquake disrupted a formerly sealed compartment of heated underground fluid, an earthquake of this magnitude and at this distance represents at most only a very minor disturbance. It is, therefore, probable that some sort of underlying process, perhaps the movement of magma underground, both triggered the earthquake and liberated the springs.

The activity at Hot Springs continues, providing a portal into the underground world whose scale and complexity challenge human imagination. Hot Springs offers but a glimpse of the caldera system. Still, the glimpse is perhaps enough to give the intrepid earthquake-volcano tourist a small sense of the immense, and clearly restless, volcanic system that lies below.

One final area remains to be explored to complete our tour of the Owens Valley. Although we have, strictly speaking, left the Owens Valley behind by the time we arrive at Long Valley, our fault- and volcano-finding tour will end at, Mono Lake.

Near the center of Mono Lake lies Paoha Island, a mostly sedimentary dome of land pushed upward, perhaps as recently as 200 years ago, by magma welling up below the surface. A darker island west of Paoha, called Negit, is a basaltic cinder cone, the remnant of an eruption approximately 1,400 years ago. Immediately northeast of the lake, we find an unusually flat-topped volcano, Black Point. Geologists speculate that Black Point may have erupted underwater at a time when the water level in Mono Lake was much higher than it is today.

Among the best-known and most-photographed features at Mono Lake are the bizarre spires known as tufa towers. Not volcanic in origin, these towers are the ghostly land relics of deposits of calcium carbonate that formed where underwater springs bearing dissolved calcium met the carbonate-rich water of the lake. Many of Mono Lake's tufa towers are visible today because the lake's water level fell dramatically after the Los Angeles Department of Water and Power began diverting water from the lake in 1941. Since that time, the water volume of the lake has decreased approximately in half, and its salinity has doubled.

At once foreboding and beautiful, Mono Lake has inspired generations of photographers, poets, and naturalists alike. After astutely deducing that the region's stark volcanic features must be young, John Muir described the Mono Lake region as, "A country of wonderful contrasts. Hot deserts bounded by snowladen mountains,—cinders and ashes scattered on glacier-polished pavements,—frost and fire working together in the making of beauty."

Although he professed a preference for the "green side of the mountains," Muir again revealed his quintessential naturalist's sensibilities in his concluding remarks about the "gray east side": "Reading these grand mountain manuscripts displayed through every vicissitude of heat and cold, calm and storm, upheaving volcanoes and down-grinding glaciers, we see that everything in Nature called destruction must be creation,—a change from beauty to beauty." Having reached Mono Lake after traveling through every vicissitude of fire and ice, there are no words more fit than these with which to end a tour of the Owens Valley and the eastern Sierra Nevada.

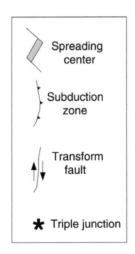

8 Finding Fault Beyond the Borders

Although clearly not defined based on geology, California's boundaries encompass a remarkably distinct geologic terrain—the transform part of the boundary between the North American and Pacific plates. The San Andreas fault is a ribbon that begins just north of the United States–Mexico border and heads offshore to its northern terminus just south of the California-Oregon border near

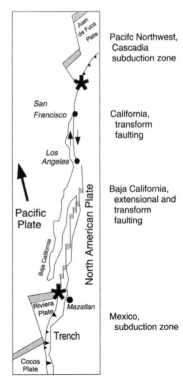

Spreading center

Subduction zone

Transform fault

★ Triple junction

Pacifc Northwest, Cascadia subduction zone

California, transform faulting

Baja California, extensional and transform faulting

Mexico, subduction zone

Juan de Fuca Plate

San Francisco

Los Angeles

Pacific Plate

North American Plate

Baja California

Riviera Plate

Mazatlan

Trench

Cocos Plate

Plate boundary along North America between the Pacific Northwest (Cascadia) subduction zone and the Mexican subduction zone

Cape Mendocino. California doesn't just have its fault systems; in a very real sense, California *is* a fault system—shaken, stirred, and carved over the ages into a landscape as dynamic as it is unique.

There is, however, life beyond the borders. South of California's border with Mexico, we first encounter a zone of spreading in the Gulf of California before reaching the great subduction zone off the western coast of southern Mexico. North of the state border, and the Mendocino Triple Junction, we find the Cascadia subduction zone. And to the east, we find the Basin and Range province, where the crust is in the long, slow process of collapse and extension associated with the prehistoric configuration of the plate boundary.

In this final chapter, we will leave California behind for a brief tour of the world beyond its borders. We obviously cannot do justice to three states and part of one country in a fraction of the space devoted to a single state. This chapter, therefore, provides only an overview of the three regions and a discussion of the geographical and geologic context of the California plate-boundary system. It will also be more of a broad-brush overview than a tour guide, although California's neighbors do provide some interesting fault- (and volcano-) finding opportunities.

The Pacific Northwest

Driving northward out of California, perhaps on I-5, we leave the San Andreas system behind and encounter one of the southernmost Cascade volcanoes before we reach the Oregon border. Looming large and easily visible from the interstate, Mount Shasta signals the beginning of a whole new tectonic terrain. The San Andreas fault ends offshore at a so-called triple junction—a place where the edges of three plates come together. The transform boundary between the North American and Pacific plates abruptly gives way to the subduction boundary between the North American and Juan de Fuca plates. This radical change in plate boundary geometry makes finding faults in the Pacific Northwest an altogether different exercise than it is in California. The key faults are much harder to find in the Pacific Northwest even though they are much larger than even the San Andreas fault itself.

Also in contrast to California, the major plate-boundary faults have not called attention to themselves with major earthquakes during the early historical era. Among the scientific community, therefore, finding faults in the Pacific Northwest has not been a matter of mapping faults directly (after major earthquakes or otherwise), but rather of applying ingenious methods to elucidate the nature of faults that lurk unseen, offshore and/or deep within the crust. These investigations involve a number of disparate approaches, including studies of those earthquakes that have struck during recorded history—and in one case, about 100 years before the arrival of settlers who kept written records.

The first settlers of European descent arrived in the Pacific Northwest in the late 1700s. They hailed from Russia and established trapping settlements along

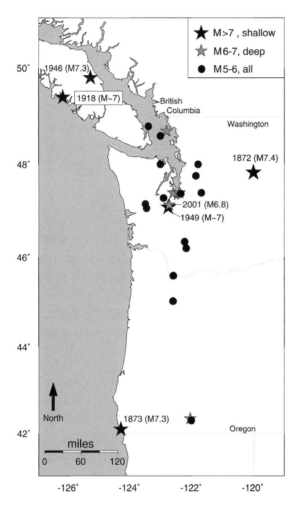

1946 (M7.3)

1918 (M~7)

British
Columbia

Washington

1872 (M7.4)

2001 (M6.8)

1949 (M~7)

North

miles

0   60   120

1873 (M7.3)

Oregon

Earthquakes in the Pacific
Northwest during recent and
recorded history

the coast as far south as northern California. Little is known, however, about earthquakes in the region in the early 1800s. Perhaps accounts remain in dusty Moscow archives, awaiting discovery by historians and modern science. But for now, our knowledge of earthquakes in the region begins in 1842, when the Oregon Trail began to bring settlers of European descent to the Pacific Northwest from points eastward. Since then, the region has experienced only a smattering of moderate to large earthquakes. One of the largest of these struck early on December 14, 1872. Accounts of the earthquake's effects clearly identify it as the largest seismic event in the Puget Sound region's recorded history—although few people were around to feel this temblor. Sparse surviving accounts describe huge landslides and ground fissures as well as a 5.5-foot-high (9-meter) geyser. (The geyser continued for several days before fading, and it left behind permanent springs.) Only a year later, a second large earthquake shook southern Oregon, a region even less densely populated than northern Washington. The 1873 earthquake was felt from Portland to San Francisco as well as aboard ships at sea. Modern estimates peg the magnitude of this earthquake at approximately 7.3, although both this value and the precise epicenter remain uncertain.

More recent earthquakes in Washington and Oregon have been more modest: the 1965 M6.5 earthquake near Renton, Washington, the 1993 M5.9 and 6.0 Klamath Falls (Oregon) earthquakes, the 1993 M5.6 Scotts Mill (Oregon) earthquake, and the 2001 M6.8 Nisqually (Seattle) earthquake. Although the largest twentieth-century events were big enough to cause damage, their moderate sizes indicate that none were truly major plate-boundary earthquakes.

Since the earliest days of the plate-tectonics revolution in the late 1960s and early 1970s, geologists have recognized the Pacific Northwest as a subduction zone. The main fault of the Cascadia subduction zone runs offshore from near the California-Oregon border to roughly the United States–Canada border, an enormous stretch of fault. Along this zone, the offshore Juan de Fuca plate sinks, or subducts, beneath the North American plate. Scientists have also recognized for some time that, by virtue of having faults whose lengths and depths are enormous, subduction zones generate the planet's largest earthquakes.

As recently as the early 1980s, scientists debated the potential of the Cascadia subduction zone to generate great earthquakes. Just as faults such as the central San Andreas sometimes move by steady creep, there are subduction zones—not many, but a few—at which subduction happens more or less steadily, without producing great earthquakes.

Although by 1980 there were few data to bear on the question, some members of the scientific community pointed cautiously to a number of the legends from the native peoples of the Pacific Northwest. Many specific legends appear to directly describe the kind of large-scale crustal motion and/or effects of tsunami that would be expected during a great subduction-triggered earthquake.

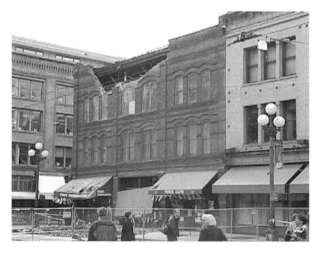

Although the 2001 Nisqually earthquake did not cause catastrophic damage, it did damage vulnerable brick and other masonry buildings such as this one in Seattle. —M. CELEBI PHOTO, U.S. GEOLOGICAL SURVEY

Ruth Ludwin, a seismologist with the University of Washington, has spent decades collecting native legends from the Pacific Northwest. Gleaned from archival sources such as diaries and published compilations, these stories resonate with richly intertwined images and themes, a unique marriage of observations of natural phenomenon and traditional lore. Kwattee, the god of creation, battles with Chief Thunderbird, who has sought to destroy the good whales of the ocean. Their struggles cause the ocean to rise and recede, sending the waters of the Pacific coursing through new channels and raising other areas up from beneath the waters. Similar themes exist in the legends of many of the region's tribes: Hoh, Quileute, and Tillamook.

Scientists are loath, however, to build scientific theory on legends, the meanings of which are subject to interpretation. Nevertheless, in the early 1980s seismologists Tom Heaton and Hiroo Kanamori took a careful look at the geologic setting of the Cascadia subduction zone. They examined factors such as the age of crust being subducted and the speed of subduction, and they concluded that the zone's properties were far closer to those of seismic subduction zones worldwide than those of the (few) aseismic ones. This was still far from compelling scientific evidence, though.

Brian Atwater:
Finding Fault from across the Ocean

Separated by the full width of the largest ocean on earth, Japan and the Pacific Northwest have become intertwined in the annals of earthquake history by virtue of tsunamis, earthquake-generated waves that traverse the Pacific with sometimes-lethal efficiency. So, perhaps it is fitting that research on prehistoric earthquakes in the Pacific Northwest has involved collaborative research by American and Japanese scientists, working on data collected on both American and Japanese soil. Brian Atwater's career reflects this symbiosis in microcosm: having found some of the earliest geologic evidence for great subduction earthquakes in the Pacific Northwest, his career later brought him to Japan, where he and Kenji Satake endeavored to interpret

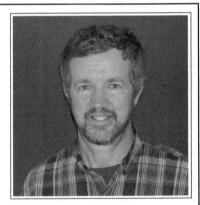

Brian Atwater

detailed ancient tsunami accounts from Japan. By interpreting accounts to obtain quantitative estimates of the height and "run-up" (inland extent) of the waves, Atwater and Satake have been able to better constrain the magnitude of the great Cascadia earthquake of January 26, 1700. It is hard to say which is more remarkable: the reward (that is, the scientific accomplishment) or the journey.

Through the 1980s, Brian Atwater of the U.S. Geological Survey and other geologists began to identify and investigate geologic evidence for tsunamis and other disruptions along the coast—evidence that pointed to large prehistoric earthquakes. Kenji Satake, then at the University of Michigan, would find the true smoking gun a dozen or so years later, in the most unlikely of possible places. Satake was analyzing a so-called orphan tsunami—that is, one without a known source—that was documented from tide gauge records in Japan on the night of January 26, 1700. Using a sophisticated modeling technique he had developed earlier and knowledge of the history of other subduction zones around the Pacific Rim, Satake concluded that the Cascadia subduction zone was the only plausible source location for this particular tsunami. This ingenious analysis provided not only the year, but also the month, day, and time of day of an earthquake that struck hundreds of years before anyone began to keep written records in the area.

Other, disparate lines of investigation corroborated Satake's conclusions. The dates of Brian Atwater's tsunami were consistent with that of Satake's orphan tsunami. An additional piece of supporting evidence came from another ingenious investigation, this one by Gordon Jacoby of Lamont-Doherty Earth Observatory and his colleagues. Jacoby analyzed tree rings from surviving trees from the "ghost forest"—coastal regions in which trees at some point suddenly found themselves

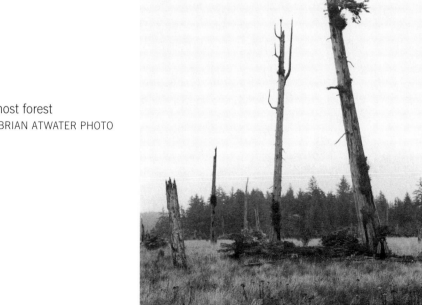

Ghost forest
—BRIAN ATWATER PHOTO

in marshy intertidal zones—and he found a sudden and marked change in their growth. By counting back from the present, this study pinpointed the time of disrupted growth to be between the growing seasons of 1699 and 1700—right on target for Satake's orphan tsunami.

By the year 2000, our understanding of the hazard the Cascadia subduction zone posed had thus grown by leaps and bounds—a rate of knowledge expansion equivalent to the scale and majesty of the subduction zone itself. The zone is approximately 600 miles (1,000 kilometers) long, stretching from the California-Oregon border to the United States–Canada border, and beyond. The so-called mega-thrust fault—the locked surface between the subducting oceanic plate and the continental one—is moreover locked over some 60 miles (100 kilometers) in depth. Were this fault to rupture stem-to-stern, as much as 38,000 square miles (100,000 square kilometers) of fault could be involved. Compare this to the biggest Big Ones expected on the San Andreas fault, which, with 300 miles (500 kilometers) of length but only about 9 miles (15 kilometers) of width, would involve a mere 2,700 square miles (7,500 square kilometers) of rupture area—a factor of about 13 times smaller. Translating this using the formulae that relate rupture area to magnitude, we find that scientists expect the Big Ones on the Cascadia subduction zone to be about a full magnitude larger than the Big Ones in California.

Californians can perhaps take a small measure of comfort from this calculation. While they face earthquakes of "only" about M8.0, our neighbors to the north face temblors in the range of M9. Throughout recorded history, the Pacific Northwest has produced fewer damaging Pretty Big Ones than has California, perhaps only a statistical fluke but perhaps the characteristic behavior of the zone. Also, many of the Pretty Big Ones, such as the 2001 Nisqually earthquake, originate deep enough that their destructive wallop is muted by the time the energy reaches the earth's surface.

Still, California cannot rightfully claim the moniker Earthquake Country all to itself. Within the United States the title belongs to the entire West Coast, as well as to Alaska.

Finding faults in the Pacific Northwest is not as easy as finding faults in California—a fact that residents of the Pacific Northwest are more than happy to point out. But, their faults are far bigger and badder than anything California has to offer. They just happen to be mainly underwater.

Even the Pretty Big Ones in the Pacific Northwest, such as Nisqually, are clearly big enough to rattle more than nerves. Moreover, evidence suggests that these events strike near the densely populated Puget Sound region. Not subduction earthquakes per se, small and moderate earthquakes along the Cascadia zone occur within the subducting slab of oceanic crust and mantle. Researchers have found that these earthquakes are caused largely by the stresses associated with

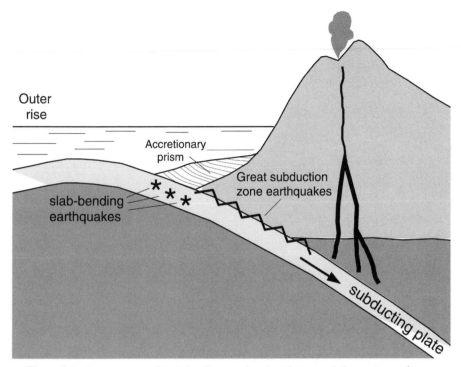

Outer rise

Accretionary prism

Great subduction zone earthquakes

slab-bending earthquakes

subducting plate

The related processes of subduction and vulcanism, and the nature of subduction-zone earthquakes. Great earthquakes originate where the subducting plate moves beneath the overriding crust. Earthquakes also occur both at shallow depths within the crust and within the sinking plate.

bending and unbending of the slab as it sinks. Although scientists do not entirely understand the distribution of such earthquakes, they appear to congregate in the Puget Sound region because the geometry of the subduction zone there is particularly complex. Along the southern Washington and north-central Oregon coasts, away from the Puget Sound region, seismologists have observed few slab-bending earthquakes.

However, a substantial additional component of hazard in the Pacific Northwest is due to faults in the continental crust, above the subduction zone. Like many of California's faults, these crustal faults are secondary in the sense that they do not reflect the main plate-boundary motion. Ultimately, however, plate boundary forces drive them, again like secondary faults in California.

In the Pacific Northwest, secondary faults provide an additional measure of hazard, compared with local plate-boundary earthquakes because some of them lie at shallow depths. The shaking from slab-bending earthquakes is muted at the surface just as ripples in a pond die away as they move outward and their energy spreads over an ever-increasing area. A Pretty Big One on a shallow crustal

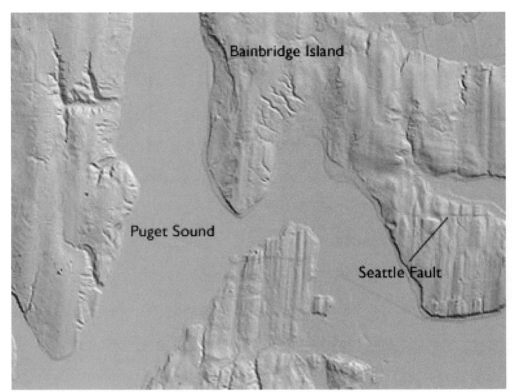

A lidar image of the Seattle region, with the extent of the Seattle fault indicated. Lidar is similar to conventional radar except that, instead of using radio waves, it employs light waves (visible, infrared, and ultraviolet). —WORK BY RALPH HAUGERUD AND DAVID HARDING

fault in the Pacific Northwest will cause damage comparable to that from a Pretty Big One in California.

One possible source zone of a Pretty Big One in the Pacific Northwest is the Seattle fault. First identified as a possible fault zone in 1965 based on detailed gravity data, the Seattle fault is a complex set of thrust faults that pass through downtown Seattle and the Puget Lowland of western Washington. Myriad factors complicate finding the fault in Seattle, including that the fault is both complex and partly underwater.

One of the primary methods for fault finding underwater involves marine surveys. In this line of attack, underwater explosions generate strong signals in the water that travel down into the underlying crust and bounce back to be recorded on special instrumentation. Conceptually, the methodology follows the approach used to study faults on dry land. Not surprisingly, however, logistics are another matter. Setting off underwater blasts might be relatively straightforward, but recording the waves requires far more involved instrumentation than similar studies on dry land. And ship time does not come cheap.

Nonetheless geologists have succeeded in obtaining increasingly refined images of the Seattle fault and a better understanding of its past and probable future behavior. Work by Tom Pratt and his colleagues, largely based on marine surveys in the 1990s, suggests that the total area of the fault is large enough to generate an earthquake as large as M7.6 to M7.7. Echoing results from secondary faults in California, researchers don't expect such earthquakes to occur commonly.

Several lines of evidence, including patterns of coastal uplift and indications of tsunamis, suggest that a large earthquake struck on the Seattle fault around 900 A.D. Available data cannot constrain the magnitude of this earthquake with precision, but they suggest a value upwards of M7.0. Whatever the magnitude, seismologists infer that the earthquake caused a tsunami in Puget Sound, landslides in Lake Washington, and rock avalanches in the Olympic Mountains—clearly a powerful event. Also echoing the situation in California, the fault appears to represent a low-probability but potentially enormous hazard. Paralleling the Los Angeles region in particular, when the next large earthquake rumbles on the Seattle fault, it will be especially damaging because of its proximity to population centers—not only closer laterally to the major population centers than the major plate-boundary fault, but also closer vertically.

Oregon has its faults as well. The state represents something of a microcosm of the West: a transect across southern Oregon crosses three distinct geologic provinces. The eastern side of the state edges into the extensional Basin and Range province, central Oregon is spanned by the Cascade volcanoes, and along the coast we find the subduction zone itself.

In addition to the 1873 earthquake in southern Oregon, notable earthquakes have struck there in more recent recorded history. These include a shock felt strongly in Portland in 1892, a damaging earthquake near the state line close to Walla Walla, Washington, in 1936, the 1993 Klamath Falls earthquakes, and a steady spattering of other events large enough to cause at least minor damage.

The 1993 M5.9 and M6.0 Klamath Falls earthquakes, both of which struck on September 20, caused two deaths and ten million dollars in property damage. The most destructive earthquake in Oregon's history, however, was the smaller M5.6 Scotts Mill earthquake on March 25, 1993. Whereas Klamath Falls is in a relatively sparsely populated part of southern Oregon, the Scotts Mills earthquake struck the more densely populated northern edge of the state. By virtue of its proximity to cities and towns, this modest temblor caused some thirty million dollars in property damage, including substantial damage to the Capitol rotunda in Salem.

In both Oregon and Washington, however, the onshore fault systems are secondary features associated with the main plate boundary fault, which is underwater. The onshore faults are therefore less pronounced, and less obvious, than the major plate-boundary faults in California. Nonetheless, even our short recorded history shows that we can expect damaging earthquakes of magnitudes approaching and possibly even exceeding 7.0. And we can look forward to much, much larger subduction zone earthquakes as well—available evidence suggests that these monster quakes hit about every 300 to 600 years, on average. (Did I mention that the last one was in 1700?)

The most spectacular points of geologic interest in both Oregon and Washington are not their faults but their volcanoes. As in California, Pacific Northwest volcanoes are important players in the plate-boundary system. Characteristic of subduction zones worldwide, a volcanic chain stretches through both Oregon and Washington, as well as northernmost California, just inboard of the subduction zone. The plate boundary itself changes character abruptly at the triple junction where the Pacific, North America, and Juan de Fuca plates meet, and the volcanic signature—an embroidery of the crust, if you will—extends over the same region. These volcanoes represent (perhaps appropriately for an ecologically minded, politically correct region) a recycling scheme of sorts, as some subducted crust makes its way back to the surface. As the slab sinks, its temperature increases, its minerals transforming as the heat and pressure rise. But some so-called volatiles heat enough to become buoyant and rise back up to the surface as magma.

The southernmost Cascade volcano, Mount Lassen in northern California, owns the distinction of being one of the two Cascade volcanoes to have erupted in the twentieth century. Part of the much larger Tehama volcanic system, which erupted hundreds of thousands of years ago, Lassen Peak experienced a series of eruptions

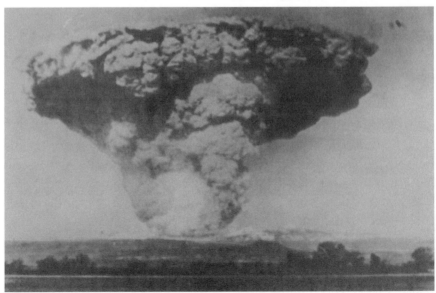

Eruption of Lassen volcano, California, in 1915.
—R. I. MEYERS PHOTO, DISTRIBUTED BY NOAA/NGDC

between 1914 and 1917. On May 22 of 1915, a blast sent ash as far east as Reno and created a zone of devastation near the mountain that can still be seen today.

We credit much of our knowledge of the 1914–1917 eruptions to the efforts of Benjamin Franklin Loomis, a local businessman and photographer. Loomis climbed to the top of Lassen Peak six times, returning with photographs and descriptions of craters and other features forming at the summit. (It is remarkable, not to mention fortunate, that he managed to avoid being blown to bits during these wanderings up and down such a ferociously active volcano.) The central crater eventually grew to some 250 yards (230 meters) by 120 to 140 yards (110 to 130 meters) across, with a depth up to 40 feet (13 meters). Loomis continued to document the prolonged period of unrest, including steam explosions in 1914–1915; a large steam explosion, an avalanche, and mudflows on May 19, 1915; the large eruption on May 22, 1915; and renewed steam eruptions in May of 1917. The descriptions and photographs Loomis left behind have allowed scientists to unravel the eruptive sequence in far greater detail than would have been possible without his efforts.

As a brief aside, you might notice that throughout this chapter the month of May features prominently. Not only the 1915 and 1917 eruptions at Lassen but also the 1980 eruption of Mount St. Helens (and the nearly coincidental onset of unrest at Long Valley caldera) took place in May. Scientists do not know of a mechanism that accounts for any general seasonality of volcanic eruptions, but the coincidences are interesting.

Among the least visited of the country's national parks, Lassen offers abundant and spectacular evidence of volcanic activity. Located 50 miles east of Redding on California 44, the park includes such notable sites as a well-graded (if not quite easy) trail to the top of Lassen Peak, as well as boiling mud pots and other active features at Devil's Kitchen and in the Bumpass Hell area. An easy, lovely trail leads hikers to Bumpass Hell, where scalding hot pools, boiling mud pots, and a pervasive sulfurous stench greet visitors—imparting an understanding of the area's Hadean connection.

Mount Saint Helens

In 1980, the world's attentions were drawn to another of the volcanoes in this chain: Mount Saint Helens in southern Washington. Although not very seismically or volcanically active, through most of the twentieth century, Mount St. Helens stirred to life on March 20, 1980, with a M4.1 earthquake below the mountain. This modest temblor marked the end of more than a century of slumber and the beginning of the end of a mountain that generations of outdoor enthusiasts had known and loved.

After its initial stirrings, Mount St. Helens wasted no time springing to life in earnest. Within four days, instruments were recording frequent earthquakes, and on March 25, U.S. Geological Survey geologist Donal Mullineaux flew to Vancouver, Washington, to lead and coordinate the investigations and response. Two days later, the mountain sent a cloud of smoke and debris more than a mile into the atmosphere, and a large new fracture opened across the top of the mountain.

Geologists recognized that the March 27 eruption, though dramatic, was small potatoes, although they differed in their predictions of future activity—both its possible timing and its size. Meanwhile, activity on the mountain escalated, setting off more minor eruptions, creating new summit craters, and producing a pronounced new bulge on the north side of the volcano. U.S. Geological Survey geologist David Johnston was among those who interpreted these signs as ominous and likely to portend a major eruption.

At the beginning of April, scientists observed their first "tremor," a characteristic sustained signal seen only at active volcanoes and generated by the underground migration of magma that precedes eruptions. Moving magma causes not only earthquakes in the crust surrounding a magma chamber or conduit, but also prolonged seismic signals associated with the magma movement itself—not unlike the hum of water coursing through pipes.

Although volcanoes sometimes produce energetic sequences of earthquakes that fade away without ado, tremors generally signal unrest that will build to eruptions. By early April the scientific community, therefore, relayed their concerns to public officials, who declared a state of emergency on April 3 and set up roadblocks staffed with National Guard personnel. Officials urged residents of the area to evacuate and most complied.

Through April and early May, the mountain seemed to play an agonizing game of cat and mouse with scientists and the public, settling down intermittently before exhibiting escalating unrest. At 8:32 on the morning of May 18, David Johnston radioed U.S. Geological Survey headquarters from his watch post 6 miles (10 kilometers) from the summit: "Vancouver . . . Vancouver . . . this is it!" These would be the last known words of the 31-year-old scientist, whose observation point proved less safe than believed when the mountain unexpectedly sent a huge lateral blast northward, in the direction of his position.

We might imagine that volcanoes merely "blow their tops," but an eruption of a volcano like Mount St. Helens is generally a prolonged and complex affair. The collapse of the mountain generated an enormous avalanche of rock and other debris that sped down the mountain at roughly 300 miles per hour, and triggered a 290-yard-high (270 meters, or nearly three football fields) wave in Spirit Lake that washed up the opposite shore and then back. By the time the dust and water had settled, the surface of the lake was carpeted by tens of thousands of trees, broken and tossed about like so many toothpicks.

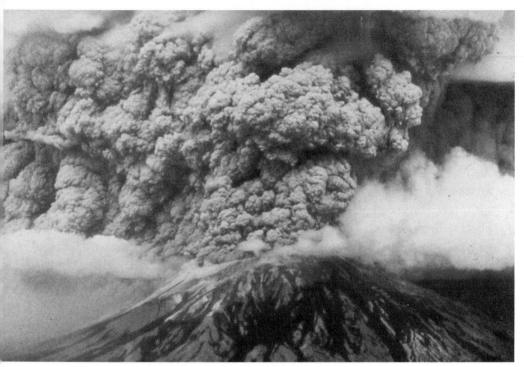

Eruption of Mount St. Helens in 1980 —DISTRIBUTED BY NOAA/NGDC

With much of the mountainside gone, the magma beneath Mt. Saint Helens was suddenly confined by far less pressure, and generated the northward blast that killed David Johnston and fifty-six other people unlucky (or foolish) enough to be in its path.

The mountain exploded at 8:32:45 A.M.; within 35 seconds it had obliterated everything within 8 miles (13 kilometers). Another 40 seconds later, the blast had flattened everything within 15 miles (25 kilometers), including enough trees to build several hundred thousand homes.

Although astonishingly violent, the initial blast from Mt. Saint Helens was not the main show. At 8:47 A.M., a vertical column of ash and steam rose 12 miles (20 kilometers) into the air above the volcano, the onset of the primary eruption. As if the drama weren't already enough, the tumultuous disruption created its own weather system, including flashes of lightning.

Ejected into the atmosphere, the ash began a remarkable journey. By 10 A.M., the ash cloud had reached Yakima, Washington, where automatic street lights registered the darkness and turned on. By the next day, the ash cloud continued to spread, reaching the central United States. Fine particles from the eruption remained detectable in the atmosphere for two full years.

The primary eruption of Mount St. Helens, which sent some 0.06 cubic miles (0.25 cubic kilometers or about 250 *million* cubic yards) of ash into the atmosphere, ended around 5:30 P.M. on May 18—fully nine hours after it had begun. During the ensuing months, it erupted several more times, although the eruptions were much smaller.

The 1980 eruptions left a meager carcass where a majestic mountain once stood. Countless photographs have been taken of the remnants of Mount St. Helens, but no two-dimensional image does justice to what the human eye sees. The view up close is staggering—and the extent to which the formerly huge and formidable mountain is now simply gone is nearly unfathomable. Eventually, though, as magma pushes up deep within the volcano and the eruptive cycle ends, the mountain will be rebuilt.

Notwithstanding the tragic loss of life and the enormous devastation the 1980 eruption caused, as natural hazards go, volcanoes are more considerate, as a rule, than earthquakes. Almost without exception through recent times, a specific pattern of earthquake activity has preceded eruptions worldwide. Although the duration and other details vary considerably from case to case, sequences invariably include an accelerated rate of earthquakes as well as the characteristic sustained signal known as tremor.

Through the late twentieth century, a burgeoning and exciting subfield of volcano seismology developed. Using seismic instruments, scientists began listening to the very heartbeat of active volcanoes and made considerable strides in identifying the nature of seismic signals generated by volcanic activity. Whereas the twentieth century saw (questionably) a single successful earthquake prediction—in Haicheng, China, in 1975—scientists successfully predicted several major eruptions. These included not only Mt. Saint Helens but also Mount Pinatubo in the Philippines in 1991 and Redoubt Volcano in Alaska in 1989, among others.

This successful track record has been a source of justifiable gratification for the "volcano cowboys" who strive to understand and ultimately predict the nature of the beast. It is not often that a scientist knows with certainty that his or her efforts have saved lives. Furthermore, the predictability of eruptions represents a good news–bad news situation for volcanologists, whose zeal to study volcanoes often lands them in front-row seats to eruptions—seats that, as in David Johnston's case, can prove deadly. If earthquake prediction ever becomes a reality, the occupational hazards of seismology will no doubt rise considerably. Being every bit as enthusiastic (if not daft) as their compatriots in volcano science, earthquake scientists will also rush to find front-row seats to impending earthquakes.

The track record of successful eruption predictions should provide a measure of comfort to those who live near volcanoes, but this measure has its limits. In 1980, less than eight weeks separated the initial rumbling from the major

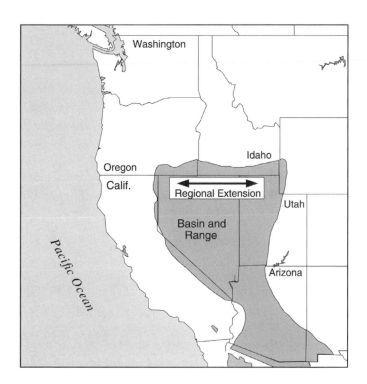

The Basin and
Range province

eruption of Mount St. Helens, and "detonation" sequences as short as a single
day have preceded eruptions of other volcanoes worldwide.

For scientists as well as residents of the region, the Cascadia subduction zone
gives rise to myriad and complex hazards, including earthquakes, volcanoes, and
tsunamis. Those who flee California for the greener pastures of the Pacific Northwest
may succeed in leaving some of the commotion behind, but sooner or later they
will discover that every place has its faults, especially along the Ring of Fire.

The Basin and Range

If we head north out of California, we leave the transform plate boundary and
encounter a subduction zone. If we leave the state to the east, we move into a
region of mainly extension—the Basin and Range province. Fault systems in the
northwest corner of Nevada represent a continuation of those found in northern
California and are therefore part of the transform plate boundary. For the most
part, however, active faults in Nevada do not reflect the forces associated with
the current plate boundary. Instead, they may represent the long-lived consequences
of subduction along the pre–San Andreas plate boundary, forces that pushed
much of western North America upward. And what goes up, must come down.
Where the earth's crust is concerned, coming down generally involves motion
on normal faults.

While Nevada is not the axis of an active plate boundary in the same way
that California is, it is part of a larger region where the forces of plate tectonics—

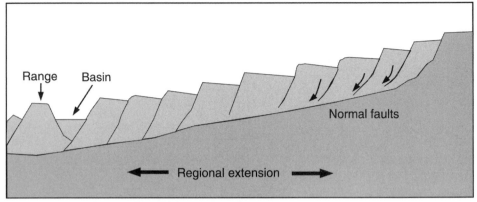

The process of normal faulting in the Basin and Range province extends the crust and creates the region's signature basins and ranges.

and faults—are active. In a sense, Nevada and its environs represent something of a transition zone between the major plate-boundary faults of the West and the much more staid and stable midcontinent.

Nevada's faults produced a number of substantial earthquakes during the twentieth century, although some are now slipping beyond the reach of memory. On the afternoon of October 2, 1915, an earthquake struck near Pleasant Valley and perceptibly shook much of northern Nevada. About two hours later, a stronger shock struck, generating perceptible ground motions over more than 200 miles. A sequence of smaller shocks, described as nearly continuous, then commenced, culminating with a main shock that created a fault scarp 5 to 9 feet (1.6 to 3 meters) high and nearly 25 miles (40 kilometers) long. The ground motions from this major temblor, of approximately M7, were felt throughout most of the state and well into California.

On December 20, 1932, another large earthquake struck, this time in west-central Nevada, again generating ground motions felt throughout the state and as far-flung as San Francisco and Los Angeles. This so-called Cedar Mountain earthquake had an estimated magnitude of 7.2. It left a complex zone of surface fissures, which revealed a mix of vertical and lateral motion, over a swath some 40 miles (63 kilometers) long and 4 to 9 miles (6 to 15 kilometers) wide. Fortunately, the epicentral region was sparsely populated at the time, so the earthquake caused very little damage despite its appreciable size. Two years later, a smaller but still substantial earthquake struck within about 50 miles of the 1932 event.

The best-known earthquakes in Nevada—the Dixie Valley earthquakes—struck near the town of Fallon in 1954, a cluster of four quakes with magnitudes of 6.6, 6.8, 7.1, and 6.8. The first three temblors happened in July, August, and December, respectively, and the fourth followed the third by just four minutes. Although probably no larger than the earlier 1915 and 1932 events, the 1954 Dixie Valley

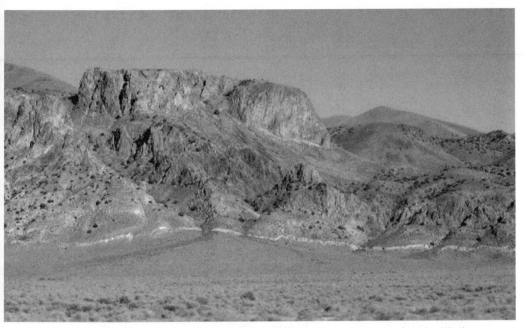

The narrow, light ribbon at the base of the hills is the scarp associated with the 1915 Pleasant Valley, Nevada, earthquake —NOAA/NGDC PHOTO

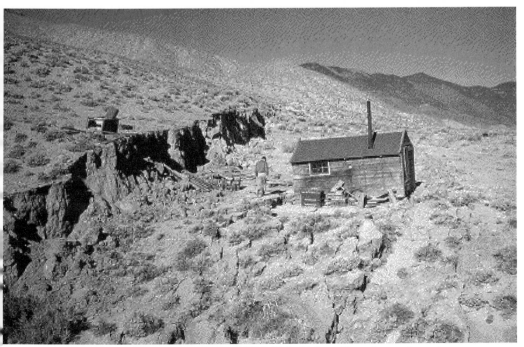

The scarp associated with the 1954 Dixie Valley, Nevada, earthquakes

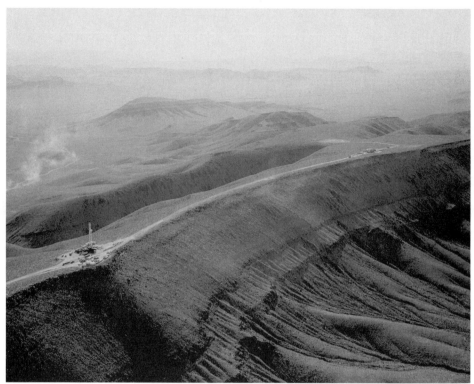
View of Yucca Mountain, the proposed high-level nuclear waste repository site —DOE PHOTO

sequence received far more attention from the scientific world simply because the geologic and seismologic communities were much larger in 1954 than they had been just a few decades earlier. Hugo Benioff, one of the founding fathers of modern seismology, was among the scientists to visit and document the substantial fault scarps these events generated.

All the large early and mid-twentieth century earthquakes in Nevada were normal faulting events, the consequences of the extensional forces that continue to stretch the Basin and Range province. Both the December 1954 earthquake and the southern tail of the July 1954 rupture cross U.S. 50, the latter about 15 miles east of Fallon and the former another 22 miles farther east. It is, however, a very long way to go (for most people) to find faults.

Although geologists at the time knew the four Dixie Valley quakes were part of the same sequence, they would not understand the evolution of the sequence until nearly half a century later. It was only in the 1990s, after researchers developed theories of stress transfer, that seismologist Gene Ichinose and his colleagues could show that the Nevada sequence was yet another case of successively toppling dominoes. Like twentieth-century earthquakes in Turkey, and perhaps like coastal southern California earthquakes since the seventeenth century, each successive Fairview Peak event was triggered by the change in stress resulting from the preceding one(s).

Although the state was a seismologically lively place for a few decades in the early twentieth century, the latter part of the century was fairly quiet. During this time, seismological interest in Nevada focused largely on a single public policy issue: the geologic suitability of the proposed high-level nuclear waste facility at Yucca Mountain in western Nevada.

Finding faults at Yucca Mountain was thus part of a multibillion dollar endeavor, quite possibly the most expensive focused geologic investigation ever conducted in the United States. In 1976, the director of the U.S. Geological Survey, Vincent McKelvey, suggested that waste be disposed of at the Nevada Test Site, testing ground for the nuclear weapons program. In 1982, the Nuclear Waste Policy Act targeted three sites for investigation, including Yucca Mountain at the western edge of the Nevada Test Site.

In 1987, Congress curtailed investigations of the other two sites, focusing their efforts on determining the suitability of Yucca Mountain. The government then funded studies to the tune of three billion dollars to investigate the site, with a goal of storing wastes there by 2010. Although government programs with billion-dollar price tags are scarcely unusual, by some measures this sum is staggering. The National Earthquake Hazards Reduction Program, which has supported much of the hazards-oriented earthquake research in the country since being enacted in 1977, has an annual budget of approximately one hundred million (inflation-adjusted) dollars. The government has therefore invested as much in Yucca Mountain as they've spent on three decades of research to mitigate earthquake hazards.

The stakes at Yucca Mountain, however, are enormous. Containment facilities will house spent fuel rods from nuclear power plants, whose uranium and plutonium will remain radioactive for millions of years. A lot of things can happen in even 50,000 years: ice ages can come and go, local climates can become wetter or more arid, and infrequent earthquakes can inflict devastation—several times over. For all we know, humans could be extinct in 50,000 years; our pollution could outlive us all. Or perhaps radioactive contamination will be the catalyst for human extinction.

Yucca Mountain is an example of a common, substantial problem in earthquake hazard assessment: the so-called low-probability, high-impact earthquake. This problem looms large in the central and eastern United States, where earthquakes are expected to strike infrequently but to have a large impact if and when they do. Nowhere is this problem as acute as it is at Yucca Mountain.

Reservations and doomsday scenarios notwithstanding, the Yucca Mountain project marches forward. The facilities are designed to withstand earthquakes expected to strike over the next 10,000 years, and it will be constructed with the best engineering current technology can provide. Yet, as U.S. Geological Survey scientist Tom Hanks conceded in a 1999 report, nobody can provide an absolute guarantee that Yucca Mountain will withstand everything the next 50,000 years might dish up.

One of the primary concerns for long-term safety at Yucca Mountain involves the seepage of groundwater. Water corrodes. The two salient questions regarding Yucca Mountain, therefore, are: how much water will the waste containers be exposed to?; and how long will it take for the storage containers to corrode? The second question is the purview of engineering, and it is all but impossible to answer. Certain metals and alloys are known to be exceptionally stable, but nuclear waste disposal involves a timescale entirely different than anything considered before. It may be beyond the capabilities of current technology to develop a container that can outlive nuclear waste.

The first question then becomes especially critical. One of the original rationales for choosing the Yucca Mountain site was that scientists thought the geologic terrain, a highly compressed volcanic ash, was impenetrable to rainfall. Digging into the mountain, however, they encountered a complex web of fissures and faults, some of which provide conduits for an abundant flow of groundwater.

Worse yet, scientists identified chlorine 36 in deep groundwater at Yucca Mountain. Chlorine 36 is an isotope that does not exist naturally and can only have been generated by nuclear bomb testing in the area. The federal government conducted the first nuclear tests at the Nevada Test Site in 1962, which implies that rainwater can find its way deep into Yucca Mountain in as little as forty years.

The debate regarding the long-term safety of Yucca Mountain thus involves far more than earthquakes, which represent only one of myriad concerns. Prior to the final decision in Washington, D.C., the state of Nevada retained the option to serve a "notice of disapproval" that, if served, would be accepted or overridden by Congress. Nevada did choose to challenge a decision by President George W. Bush to move forward with plans; but in 2002, Congress overruled the challenge. State officials and residents have long harbored concerns about the safety of Yucca Mountain given both the groundwater issues and that Nevada is the third most seismically active state in the contiguous United States. Native Pauite and western Shoshone tribes raised their voices in protest as well, pointing to sacred sites and artifacts on the mountain, access to which was impossible even during the investigation stage.

NIMBY (Not In My Backyard) protests have become commonplace in the West, but in western Nevada these protests seem more than justified, given that the area is part of the extended active plate-boundary region. In recent times, earthquake activity has clustered in north-central Nevada, but scientists now believe this cluster to be something of a fluke. That is, the earthquakes through the first half of the twentieth century appear to have followed like a cascade of dominoes once the first large event happened to strike. If so, northern Nevada is not expected to be especially active over the long haul; it was merely the site of the most recent cluster. The next cluster in the state could well be elsewhere. Such clusters seem to pop up and fade away on long timescales. Recall that the Mojave Desert faults discussed in chapter 6 have sprung to life only once every 10,000 years or so. This is a small measure of comfort, given the timescales of concern at Yucca Mountain.

Proponents of the Yucca Mountain site point out that some 70,000 metric tons of high-level nuclear waste are already squirreled away at more than a hundred sites throughout the United States, each unquestionably designed to far less exacting standards than Yucca Mountain facilities will be. Some of the sites are moreover near major population centers, some of which are exposed to significant earthquake hazard. We have developed nuclear weapons and now rely on nuclear energy, they argue; the waste has to go somewhere.

In 2002, the Nuclear Waste Technical Review Board, a panel of eleven independent experts appointed by Congress, concluded that the government's case for building the Yucca Mountain facility was "weak to moderate." Not exactly a ringing endorsement—or one that inspires confidence in mankind's long-term stewardship of the planet. But with no other options on the table—and with the status quo so worrisome in its own right—"weak to moderate" appears to be the best we can do.

Finding Fault South of the Border

The California plate boundary continues south of the border, a direct and yet indirect continuation of the San Andreas fault. The transition between transform—that is, right-lateral strike-slip movement—and spreading begins before the fault leaves California. A significant component of extension gives rise to recent volcanic activity beneath and south of the southern Salton Sea. The Salton Sea, formerly the Salton Trough, is steadily sinking as a consequence of the ongoing process of extension.

The border region is truly transitionary. Not only does some extension lap north of the border, but some of California's strike-slip faults continue south of the border as well. The Imperial fault, a strike-slip fault that ruptured in 1940 and again in 1979 (see chapter 6) extends well south of the border. So, too, do the coastal fault systems (see chapter 3) extend into northern Baja California. Tom Rockwell and his colleagues have found evidence for a large earthquake on the Agua Blanca fault within 160 years of A.D. 1640. This fault skirts the Baja California coast, remaining just offshore some 60 miles (100 kilometers) south of the border before coming back onto land.

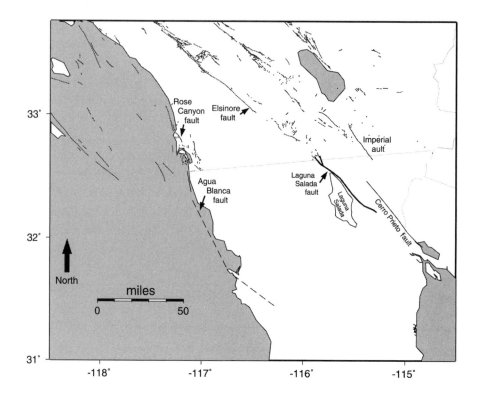

Faults in California and Baja California, Mexico

The dates of earthquakes that researchers identify with paleoseismology techniques are never precise and are typically known only to within a few decades (sometimes a century or two) because of the inherent limitations of the method as well as imprecision in dating techniques (usually carbon-14). Evidence assembled to date indicates that both the Agua Blanca and the Rose Canyon faults ruptured in large earthquakes between about 1500 and 1800, with most probable dates in both cases around 1640 to 1650. These two earthquakes could therefore be one and the same—that is, one very large combined rupture on both faults. Or they could have happened anywhere from a few hours to 100 years apart. This type of ambiguity arises very commonly in paleoseismology, and it represents one of the biggest challenges associated with the method: connecting the dots.

Nonetheless, researchers have little doubt that the faults themselves are connected, both in the Imperial Valley region and along the coast of southern California and northern Baja California. Neither faults nor earthquakes care one whit about political boundaries.

For the most part, however, California and Mexico represent very different tectonic regimes, and the effects of extension are far more manifest below the border. Not too far south into northern Mexico, the lateral component of plate motion peters out, giving way to a mixed zone with both lateral and extensional forces. The extensional forces are slowly but inexorably stripping Baja California away from the rest of Mexico. Here again, finding fault outside of California requires that we look underwater, a task that is not easy for the professional earth scientist and all but impossible for the amateur earthquake tourist.

One of the major faults in northern Baja California is the Laguna Salada fault, which appears to have ruptured during the 1892 Laguna Salada earthquake. This temblor was centered in an essentially uninhabited part of Baja California at a time when regional population density was low as well. Because only sparse data are available to map out the distribution of shaking, magnitude estimates of this earthquake have varied wildly. By some accounts, it was among the largest earthquakes to have ever struck in California and Baja California. More recent estimates, however, peg it at about M7.2—not a great earthquake but still a major event. Shaking was severe enough to cause alarm 75 miles (125 kilometers) away in San Diego and to destroy adobe buildings at the Carrizo stage depot in San Diego County. In Los Angeles the ground motions were large enough to cause panic, but no damage was reported.

Laguna Salada itself is a lagoon (the literal translation is "salt lake") within a basin created by offsets in the Laguna Salada fault system. Geologists have mapped the Laguna Salada fault for some 60 miles (100 kilometers), skirting along the eastern shore of Laguna Salada. To the east-southeast of Laguna Salada fault is the Cerro Prieto fault. This fault is part of the Cerro Prieto spreading center, which extends south through the Gulf of California.

Earthquake hazard in Baja California extends from stem to stern. According to local lore, earthquakes have taken a toll in the oldest town in Baja California, Loreto, 90 miles (140 kilometers) south of Mulegé. In 1697, the Jesuits founded Loreto, known for incomparable scenery both on land and offshore. They built the mission of Nuestra Señora de Loreta in 1752, and it has been rebuilt many times following damaging earthquakes, hurricanes, and floods. Reliable early earthquake catalogs from the region are difficult to find, but in the town of La Paz, farther toward the southern tip of Baja California, significant earthquakes have struck in more recent times, including a M6.2 earthquake and M5.6 aftershock on June 30, 1995.

Continuing farther south along the Mexico border, we find that the zone of extension is limited. Not far south of the southern end of Baja California, we encounter another triple junction, the meeting point of the Pacific, North American, and Cocos plates. Along the coast of Mexico south of the triple junction, the boundary between the Pacific and Cocos plates is a subduction zone that extends along the coast of Mexico and most of Central America. Taking a larger view of the Pacific Rim, California and Baja California are, to a large extent, aberrations—

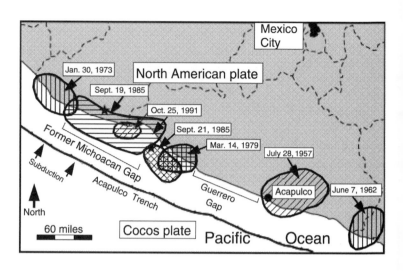

Recent large subduction zone earthquakes in Mexico —FROM WORK BY JOHN ANDERSON AND OTHERS

small snippets of transform and extensional plate boundary in a ring of great subduction zones. Making the circuit counterclockwise from the Pacific Northwest, we find a veritable hit parade of famous subduction zones: Alaska, Japan, the South Pacific, South America, and Mexico. Think for a moment about the region's moniker, the Ring of Fire, which reflects not earthquakes but rather the numerous active volcanoes, such as those in Cascadia, that rise just inboard from the subduction zones around the Pacific Rim.

We might imagine an enormous spreading center in the middle of the Pacific Ocean, churning out all of the crust that gets swallowed at the continental boundaries. In fact, while a long spreading ridge nearly bisects the Atlantic Ocean over most of its vast extent, the Pacific Ocean is underlaid by a coherent plate. In the Pacific, crust is generated in some locations along spreading centers such as the East Pacific Rise, which extends southward from the Pacific–North American–Cocos triple junction, and the Juan de Fuca Ridge in the Pacific Northwest. For the most part, though, the oceanic crust that subduction is swallowing up along the Pacific Rim is material that has underlaid oceans for a very long time. The vast Pacific Ocean is getting progressively smaller—which probably comes as small consolation to people who have endured the interminable transpacific flight.

The subduction and volcanism around the edges of the Pacific plate are similar in style, if not in fine detail, to those in the Pacific Northwest. All the subduction zones along the Pacific Rim, therefore, face the same double whammy of earthquake and volcano hazard.

Over the years, researchers have studied well the subduction zone along the west coast of Mexico, and there is little doubt as to its earthquake potential. Although subduction zones generate the biggest earthquakes on earth, all subduction zones are not created equal. In particular, some appear to be segmented on a finer scale than others and therefore generate relatively smaller earthquakes. Unlike the South American and Alaskan subduction zones, which can (and have) generated earthquakes with magnitudes as large as 9.0, the Mexican subduction zone has, at least in recent memory, generated a fairly steady, long-term smattering of earthquakes with magnitudes close to 8.0. If that's the good news, the bad news is that these more modest temblors (if a M8.0 earthquake can ever be called modest) happen more frequently than do bigger earthquakes on less segmented subduction zones.

In the early 1970s, scientist Lynn Sykes and his colleagues laid out the fundamental principles of seismic gap theory. Seismic gap theory, while not an earthquake prediction method per se, represents a fairly fundamental tenet of earthquake hazard assessments: along major plate boundaries, earthquakes are more likely to occur on segments that have not been broken in some time. As with so many things in science—and life—the devil resides in the details, and seismic gap theory has been the subject of considerable debate in earth-science circles in recent decades. Some evidence suggests that great earthquakes tend to cluster in time, such that we might expect future earthquakes to occur close to where they have occurred in the past—if not on precisely the same stretch of fault. Still, as a first-order principal, the reasoning behind seismic gap theory appears valid. Most earth scientists would, therefore, give a higher probability of a future great earthquake on the southernmost segment of the San Andreas fault, which has not ruptured for more than three hundred years, to one on the northern segment, which ruptured in 1906.

In 1981, Karen McNally and Bernard Minster focused on the history of great earthquakes on the Mexican subduction zone and observed that while most of the zone had ruptured during the twentieth century, a few conspicuous segments, or gaps, remained unbroken. They identified one particular gap as especially ripe: the so-called Guerrero gap, which stretches some 120 miles (200 kilometers) along the coast northwest of Acapulco. This work provided the impetus for the deployment of strong-motion instruments along the coast—instruments designed to record on-scale ground motions from large earthquakes. A team led by John Anderson at Scripps Institution of Oceanography began installation of this array in 1984.

The deployment, along with seismic gap theory, was apparently vindicated on the morning of September 19, 1985, when the M8.1 Michoacan earthquake struck near Acapulco. However, detailed analysis of recordings of the earthquake, including data from the local array, revealed that the temblor had ruptured the plate-boundary segment immediately northwest of the Guerrero gap. On October 9, 1995, the M7.9 Manzanillo earthquake ruptured within the Jalisco gap, the subduction zone segment northwest of the Michoacan segment. As of 2002, the Guerrero gap—originally targeted as the most ripe to produce a major temblor—

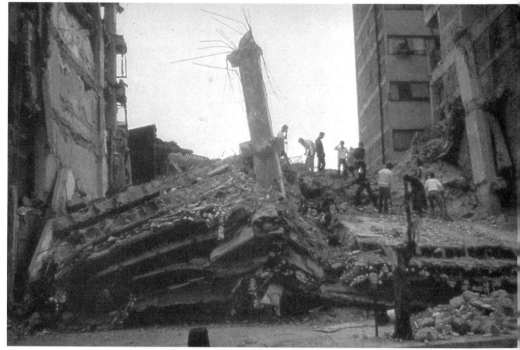

Damage in Mexico City caused by the 1985 Michoacan
earthquake —NOAA/NGDC PHOTOGRAPH

remains unbroken, and menacing. When this segment of the zone ruptures, scientists expect the effects will be similar to those in 1985.

The Guerrero gap, therefore, continues to be of tremendous concern. To most people, the 1985 Michoacan earthquake is best known for the devastation it caused several hundred miles away, when the former lake-bed zone that underlies Mexico City jiggled like a huge pan of Jell-O and didn't stop jiggling for many long seconds. By virtue of the frequency of the local shaking, which involved waves that moved from peak to trough and back to their peak in about two seconds, buildings close to twenty stories were hardest hit. Horrific images of these collapses were beamed around the world. In the end, the earthquake claimed more than 10,000 lives in Mexico City.

The coast of Mexico suffered substantial damage as well, although not the degree of devastation one might have expected. To a large extent, minimal coastal damage reflected the paucity of vulnerable buildings along the coast—especially modern high-rises such as those in Mexico City. Increasing evidence suggests, however, that compared with crustal earthquakes, at least some subduction earthquakes rupture more smoothly and more slowly, therefore releasing less destructive energy than crustal earthquakes of comparable size.

We must, however, note several caveats. First, earthquakes of M8 to M9.5 are still enormously powerful, and they clearly pose a substantial danger, particularly to vulnerable structures. Second, subduction zones are scarcely immune from the hazard earthquake sequences pose, including potentially damaging aftershocks. On January 13, 2001, a M7.6 earthquake struck offshore of El Salvador. It was followed a month later by a M6.6 earthquake on shore, some 51 miles (85 kilometers) from the January 13 shock. The main shock claimed more than eight hundred lives and more than 100,000 homes. Although much smaller, the second event caused substantial damage to nearby towns and villages, some of which were buried by huge landslides. Were a Guerrero subduction earthquake to be followed by a similar secondary shock, it could strike very close to either Acapulco or Ixtapa.

Thus does the Mexican subduction zone represent a zone of complex and substantial hazard for both coastal regions and for the twenty-million-plus inhabitants of Mexico City. Moreover, seismic gaps south of Guerrero pose a significant hazard for southern cities such as Oaxaca and Salina Cruz.

If we stand back to review Mexico from a broader tectonic perspective, we see that the offshore subduction zone fundamentally drives its current tectonics, much like the situation in both South America and the Pacific Northwest. Where Mexican and American tectonics meet, we find the exception to the rule: zones of active extension and transform faulting within a ring primarily defined by subduction.

Although scientists originally mapped these zones as separate features, they have increasingly recognized connections between the fault systems north and south of the border: the Agua Blanca and Rose Canyon faults; the Laguna Salada and Elsinore faults; and the Imperial fault, on which earthquake rupture tore straight through the border in 1940. Curiously—or perhaps not—these scientific realizations have paralleled growing trends toward cultural unity. Mexican culture has made, and continues to make, an indelible mark on California since its earliest recorded history.

In recent times, however, California has been increasingly inclined to celebrate its status not as a melting pot but rather as a stew pot, one in which different elements contribute to the flavor and texture of the whole while still maintaining individual cultural identity. The stew-pot model has clearly brought its own tensions: racial, cultural, and socioeconomic. But California remains an exercise in multiculturalism unlike any other, one whose obvious failures should not detract from its not insubstantial successes.

And it is on this note that we arrive at the end of our tour of the Golden State and its environs. California's many seemingly disparate faults are manifest, and have been so since the earliest days of the state's recorded history. Increasingly, however, scientists have recognized these faults to be part of an integrated system, not only throughout the state but also beyond the borders. This book, as the astute reader has surely long-since realized, is not simply a tour guide of California's faults but rather a celebration of them. Earthquakes scare us, and rightly so; a healthy respect for hazard impels us to take steps to mitigate risk. But the state is an extraordinary place, in almost any sense of the word, and what is bad about California is inexorably linked with what is good. California's faults define not only the state's skeleton but also its heart and soul. And so an interesting thing happens when we set out to find fault in California and to understand its place in a dynamic world: at the end of an inherently deconstructionist journey, we arrive at a newfound appreciation for the state as a whole—for all of its beauty, for all of its grandeur, for all of its faults.

Suggested Reading
and Resources

Geology of California

Sharp, Robert P., and Allen F. Glazner. 1997. *Geology Underfoot in Death Valley and Owens Valley.* Missoula, Mont.: Mountain Press.

———. 1993. *Geology Underfoot in Southern California.* Missoula, Mont.: Mountain Press.

Collier, Michael. 1999. *A Land in Motion: California's San Andreas Fault.* Berkeley: University of California Press.

Alt, David, and Donald W. Hyndman. 2000. *Roadside Geology of Northern and Central California.* Missoula, Mont.: Mountain Press.

Wallace, Robert, ed. 1990. *The San Andreas Fault System.* U.S. Geological Survey Professional Paper 1515.

Earthquakes

Bolt, Bruce A. 1999. *Earthquakes,* 5th edition. New York: W. H. Freeman and Company.

Hough, Susan Elizabeth. 2002. *Earthshaking Science: What We Know (and Don't Know) about Earthquakes.* Princeton: Princeton University Press.

Yeats, Robert S. 1998. *Living with Earthquakes in the Pacific Northwest.* Corvallis: Oregon State University Press.

———. 2001. *Living with Earthquakes in California: A Survivor's Guide.* Corvallis: Oregon State University Press.

Sieh, Kerry and Simon LeVay. 1999. *The Earth in Turmoil: Earthquakes, Volcanoes, and Their Impact on Humankind.* New York: W. H. Freeman and Company.

Kious, W. J. and R. I. Tilling. 1996. *This Dynamic Earth.* U.S. Geological Survey. (*see also* http://pubs.usgs.gov/publications/text/dynamic.html

Detailed Fault Maps

The definitive references for a detailed map trace of the San Andreas fault and a few other faults in California are the so-called strip maps published by the U.S. Geological Survey. These include the three listed below. Active fault maps of California can also be obtained from the California Geological Survey (*see* Web address below).

Brown, Robert D. 1970. *Map showing recently active breaks along the San Andreas and related faults between the northern Gabilan Range and Cholame Valley, California.* U.S. Geological Survey Miscellaneous Geologic Investigations Map I-575.

Ross, Donald C. 1976. *Map showing recently active breaks along the San Andreas fault between Tejon Pass and Cajon Pass, Southern California.* U.S. Geological Survey Miscellaneous Geologic Investigations Map I-553.

Vedder, J. G. and Robert E. Wallace. 1970. *Map showing recently active breaks along the San Andreas and related faults between Cholame Valley and Tejon Pass, California.* U.S. Geological Survey Miscellaneous Geologic Investigations Map I-574.

Web Resources

www.findingfault.com Photos from this book in living color.

www.usgs.gov. The U.S. Geological Survey's home page; abundant information about earthquakes, faults, and all things geologic.

http://earthquake.usgs.gov. Up-to-date information about earthquakes in the United States and worldwide.

http://earthquake.usgs.gov/regional/sca/ U.S. Geological Survey Southern California Earthquake Hazards Web site.

http://pasadena.wr.usgs.gov/office/hough. This author's home page—come visit!

http://pasadena.wr.usgs.gov/shake/ca. Interactive Web site allows visitors to fill out a brief questionnaire to describe the effects of a felt earthquake ("Did You Feel It?")

www.scec.org. Home page of the Southern California Earthquake Center.

www.scec.org/wallacecreek/ A virtual tour of Wallace Creek.

www.consrv.ca.gov/cgs/ Home page of the California Geological Survey.

sepwww.stanford.edu/oldsep/joe/fault_images/BayAreaSanAndreasFault.html. The San Andreas fault in the San Francisco Bay Area.

www.sfmuseum.org/ Virtual museum of the city of San Francisco contains accounts and other information about the 1906 earthquakes and other earthquakes in the San Francisco area.

www.ngdc.noaa.gov/products/ngdc_slides.html. The Web site for the National Geophysical Data Center offers slide sets of earthquakes for a nominal fee.

Index

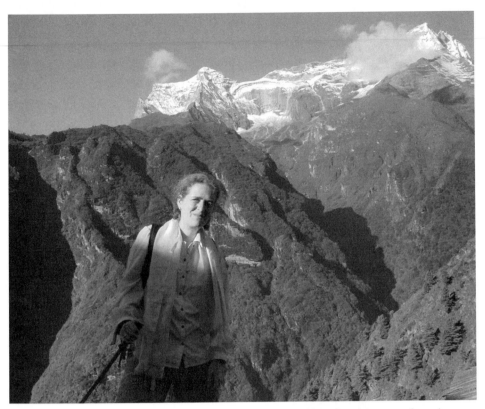

Susan Elizabeth Hough near the village of Namche, Nepal, a long way from home

About the Author

A Californian for most of her adult life, Susan Elizabeth Hough has a deep affection for the natural wonders of her adopted home state. She holds a Ph.D. in earth sciences from Scripps Institution of Oceanography at U.C. San Diego. A geophysicist with the U.S. Geological Survey in Pasadena, she studies earthquake hazards in California and historic earthquakes in the central United States and India. Hough has written many articles—both technical and popular—about earthquakes for journals, newspapers, and magazines, and she is the author of *Earthshaking Science: What We Know (and Don't Know) About Earthquakes* (Princeton University Press). She lives in southern California, just a stone's throw from the Raymond fault.

We encourage you to patronize your local bookstore. Most stores will order any title they do not stock. You may also order directly from Mountain Press, using the order form provided below or by calling our toll-free, 24-hour number and using your VISA, MasterCard, Discover or American Express.

Some geology titles of interest:

____	ROADSIDE GEOLOGY OF ALASKA	18.00
____	ROADSIDE GEOLOGY OF ARIZONA	18.00
____	ROADSIDE GEOLOGY OF S. BRITISH COLUMBIA	Can. $25.00 / U.S. 20.00
____	ROADSIDE GEOLOGY OF COLORADO, 2nd Edition	20.00
____	ROADSIDE GEOLOGY OF HAWAII	20.00
____	ROADSIDE GEOLOGY OF IDAHO	20.00
____	ROADSIDE GEOLOGY OF INDIANA	18.00
____	ROADSIDE GEOLOGY OF MAINE	18.00
____	ROADSIDE GEOLOGY OF MASSACHUSETTS	20.00
____	ROADSIDE GEOLOGY OF MONTANA	20.00
____	ROADSIDE GEOLOGY OF NEBRASKA	18.00
____	ROADSIDE GEOLOGY OF NEW MEXICO	18.00
____	ROADSIDE GEOLOGY OF NEW YORK	20.00
____	ROADSIDE GEOLOGY OF NORTHERN and CENTRAL CALIFORNIA	20.00
____	ROADSIDE GEOLOGY OF OHIO	24.00
____	ROADSIDE GEOLOGY OF OREGON	16.00
____	ROADSIDE GEOLOGY OF PENNSYLVANIA	20.00
____	ROADSIDE GEOLOGY OF SOUTH DAKOTA	20.00
____	ROADSIDE GEOLOGY OF TEXAS	20.00
____	ROADSIDE GEOLOGY OF UTAH	20.00
____	ROADSIDE GEOLOGY OF VERMONT & NEW HAMPSHIRE	14.00
____	ROADSIDE GEOLOGY OF VIRGINIA	16.00
____	ROADSIDE GEOLOGY OF WASHINGTON	18.00
____	ROADSIDE GEOLOGY OF WISCONSIN	20.00
____	ROADSIDE GEOLOGY OF WYOMING	18.00
____	ROADSIDE GEOLOGY OF THE YELLOWSTONE COUNTRY	12.00
____	FINDING FAULT IN SOUTHERN CALIFORNIA: An Earthquake Tourist Guide	18.00
____	GEOLOGY OF THE LAKE SUPERIOR REGION	22.00
____	GEOLOGY OF THE LEWIS & CLARK TRAIL IN NORTH DAKOTA	18.00
____	GEOLOGY UNDERFOOT IN CENTRAL NEVADA	16.00
____	GEOLOGY UNDERFOOT IN DEATH VALLEY AND OWENS VALLEY	16.00
____	GEOLOGY UNDERFOOT IN ILLINOIS	15.00
____	GEOLOGY UNDERFOOT IN NORTHERN ARIZONA	18.00
____	GEOLOGY UNDERFOOT IN SOUTHERN CALIFORNIA	14.00
____	GEOLOGY UNDERFOOT IN SOUTHERN UTAH	18.00

Please include $3.50 for 1-4 books, $5.00 for 5 or more books to cover shipping and handling.

Send the books marked above. I enclose $_____

Name_____

Address_____

City/State/Zip_____

☐ Payment enclosed (check or money order in U.S. funds)

Bill my: ☐ VISA   ☐ MasterCard ☐ Discover ☐ American Express

Card No._____Expiration Date_____

Security No._____ Signature_____

MOUNTAIN PRESS PUBLISHING COMPANY
P.O. Box 2399 • Missoula, MT 59806 • Order Toll-Free 1-800-234-5308
E-mail: info@mtnpress.com • Web: www.mountain-press.com